MW00436737

For We Speak of Living
A Journey Through Breast Cancer

TERESA RENDA CARLSON

FOREWORD BY LICIA CARLSON

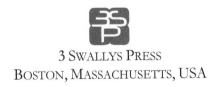

3 SWALLYS PRESS
BOSTON, MASSACHUSETTS, USA

Copyright © 2013 by Teresa Renda Carlson
First Edition 2013
All rights reserved

Paperback ISBN 978-0-9882300-2-6

To my beloved Thomas
And my precious Licia

The way is to the destructive element submit yourself,
and with the exertions of your hands and feet in the water make the
deep, deep sea keep you up.

Joseph Conrad

Contents

Foreword

Reading this book again, more than 40 years after having lived through my mother's illness, is an experience that is difficult to put into words. I am seized by a sense of profound gratitude for the remarkable fact that my mother is still here with me, that she has survived four decades in the face of a devastating diagnosis and prognosis. I am also filled with so much love for our precious family of three that she so lovingly describes, and reminded of how beautifully the three of us held each other up during these turbulent storms. The seeds sown then continue to bloom, and my parents' continued love now encircles my own little family of three.

My mother's journey through breast cancer has also been my journey. The specter of her loss haunted my childhood, though it is a testament to her wisdom that I do not remember it that way. Her positive love of life and her ability to embrace and take joy in every moment gilded my own childhood with laughter, light, color, joy, and love. Her stunning beauty and self-assurance in a body without breasts shaped my own understanding of what it means to be beautiful, to be a complete woman. And if philosopher Gareth Matthews is right that "philosophy is an adult attempt to deal with the genuinely baffling questions of childhood," encountering the harsh realities of illness and the unthinkable prospect of losing a mother at such an early age may explain my choice of profession. I am sure that these early experiences had something to do with why I was drawn to philosophy as an undergraduate, and why I now enjoy reflecting with my students on the nature of human finitude, the meaning of the good life, the power and authority of medicine, and the lines we draw between normal and abnormal, able and disabled, sick and healthy.

The 16th-century French essayist Michel de Montaigne wrote that we must befriend death, treat death as a constant companion rather than fleeing from it, so as not to live in fear of death. In many ways, mortality and cancer have been with me since I can remember. I was only 18 months the first time my mother had breast cancer, and age six the second. As she writes so beautifully in the book, my mother folded me into her own experiences of grief, sadness, fear, and joy with care and love. I have a few distinct memories of this experience: doing exercises with her, our arms crawling up the wall in unison like two little snails, slowly, and for her, painfully; her "turtles," as I called them—the two prostheses, whose presence was constant and normal, both on her body when I would hug them along with her, and on their resting place—the chair next to her bed—every evening; and her expressions of gratitude that marked every milestone, every precious event of mine that she was there to witness. I don't remember feeling fear as a child, though as I read the pages of her book, I imagine it must have been there. It resurfaced as a kind of familiar stranger many years later, when she went through two heart attacks and her third bout of cancer, but by that time I was an adult and the texture of my fears were very different from what they must have been when I was young.

Reading her book now, as a grown mother with her own child, I am also struck by how much has changed since she wrote it. Treatments for many forms of cancer have multiplied and improved tremendously, and the prognosis for so many today is nowhere near as dire as it was for my mother then. Research continues to move forward, and advances in genetics may prove to be lifesaving for cancer patients in the future. Beyond the medical world, the public face of cancer has changed significantly. Whereas in the early 1970s cancer was a taboo subject, and there were few opportunities for women to publicly share their experiences, today the cancer patient is far less stigmatized and marginalized. A myriad of cancer stories are being told in every conceivable form, by the famous and the unknown alike. While there is no question that all of these changes have been positive, these conversations, developments, and medical advances are also accompanied by new kinds of questions and challenges.

The silence that shrouded cancer during my mother's early experiences was difficult for many reasons that she outlines in her book; yet that same silence shielded me from it in many ways. As a child, my own encounters with cancer were mediated by my loving parents who, in their wisdom, decided when, where, and how to invite this unwelcome guest into my young life. Today, things are very different for children whose parents face cancer or who, themselves, are diagnosed with this disease. Signs of cancer are ubiquitous, ranging from pink ribbons and pink merchandise, charity walks and runs, celebrity profiles, TV storylines, movies, and a host of books ranging from memoirs, patient guides, and health resources. As a young child, I clung to the classic children's book *Are You My Mother?* as a way of confronting my sense of loss and alienation in the strange world of illness; today children can read books like *When Mommy Had a Mastectomy* that speak directly to the experience. The amount of information about cancer has also increased exponentially online, where there are literally millions of websites that are available at the click of a button. What is the impact of having access to so much information, particularly for children? A recent study of children between the ages of 6 and 12 who had a parent with cancer found that their access to knowledge about cancer increased their fears about both the disease itself and the loss of a parent.

Though many of the challenges my mother faced as a parent remain, the landscape parents and children encounter today is very different, shaped by new difficulties in deciding how best to help children navigate the vast quantities of information and images that shape the world of cancer. One of the reasons I believe that my mother's book is so valuable is that in telling her story from many decades ago, readers can temporarily distance themselves from the "cancerland" of today (as Barbara Ehrenreich calls it), find both resonances and differences between Teresa's story and their own, and return to the present with a new perspective.

In addition to the plethora of voices speaking about cancer today, another change that has radically transformed the experience of cancer is the advent of genetic testing. I have had to confront cancer again as an adult in a new guise, in the question of whether to get tested for the BRCA1 and BRCA2 mutations. In facing this decision, I meet cancer, not in the form of an actual disease, a concrete presence to be contended with, but as a possibility, a statistical risk expressed in probabilities. While the possibility of getting tested holds significant promise, particularly for women who have a family history of breast cancer, the decision comes with its own struggles and new species of fear, anxiety, and responsibility for both parents and children. We now have both cancer survivors and *previvors*, the term given to women who are at high risk, and who, in many cases, opt for preventative mastectomies and hysterectomies in response to a positive genetic test result.

In 1978, Susan Sontag began her book about TB and cancer, *Illness as Metaphor*, like this: "Illness is the night-side of life, a more onerous citizenship. Everyone who is born holds dual citizenship, in the kingdom of the well and in the kingdom of the sick. Although we all prefer to use only the good passport, sooner or later each of us is obliged, at least for a spell, to identify ourselves as citizens of that other place." In the 21st century, we have an intermediary kingdom, a purgatory in a sense: the category of being "at risk." The individual who occupies this place in the liminal space *between* these two worlds of health and illness holds a distinctly new kind of citizenship, a genetic passport that, as genetic testing becomes more common in the coming years, all of us may be expected to acquire.

So it is within this radically different world, amidst the thousands of other cancer books, illness narratives, self-help books, clinical guides, movies, novels, and poems, that this little gem of a book emerges, written with such honesty, immediacy, and love, this story of one young mother grappling with faith, family, and finitude. What is remarkable is that Teresa is still here to tell her story, and that we are able to hear it in her voice of those many years ago. Much has changed, and yet perhaps very little has as well. I cannot speak to how others will receive it, but for me this book is a gift, as a daughter, a mother, a woman, and as a child who has not outgrown the comfort of her mother's sweet embrace.

Licia Carlson, PhD
July 2013

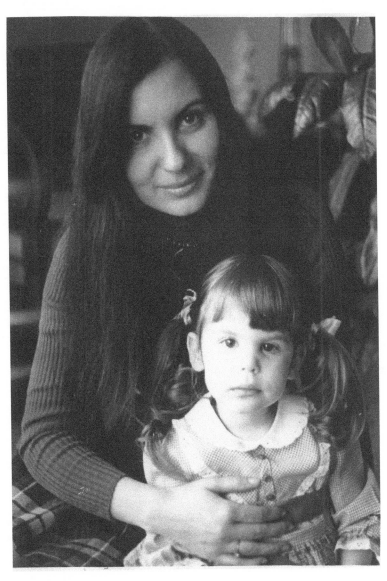

Teresa and Licia, 1972

Introduction

For one week, Teresa Carlson and I shared a room.

My surgery was over. Somehow I knew that much. I felt the motion as I was wheeled down the hall. My husband was holding my hand. Everything hurt, and I sank back into anesthetic apathy.

Later, I felt a presence in the room. Through the fog I was able to see the back of a slim girl dressed in a silky green tunic with very short pants. She was reaching to put something on a shelf. Her black hair hung in a thick swath down her back. She was small and elegant, with long lovely legs.

What was she doing here? Too young. Too healthy. Too everything. Miserably, I shut my eyes again.

Late in the afternoon I woke again and she came over to say hello.

"How are you feeling?"

"Not too bad." I tried to focus on her. What a beautiful smile. "Why are you here?" I mumbled.

She touched her breast with one finger. "A lump," she said softly.

I wanted to respond but was too fuzzy-headed, and I drifted off again. But that evening the anesthesia wore off and we embarked upon a conversation that still continues. She told me that she was 29. I was 56. She had come from Italy to Canada 10 years earlier. There she met an attractive young lawyer; they fell in love, married, and had a beautiful daughter, now 17 months old. Joy shone in her face as she told me about their life together.

Could an unexpected little concentration of cells in her breast interfere with the magic of the storybook romance? Unthinkable.

That night Teresa found herself immersed in a last-minute effort to give away some highly prized opera tickets. The Metropolitan Opera Company was scheduled for a week's engagement in Detroit, and the Carlsons had planned to attend every performance, and also to go to the late supper with the artists on opening night. What a blow to miss this beautiful experience! Teresa had lived with such music daily in Italy. Opera tunes are sung by anyone who has a voice, and the stories are as familiar as our folk tales. Traveling companies performed the great works in the smaller cities, and whole families attended.

Here in the Midwest, opera is not so available. But Teresa did not spend time bemoaning her disappointment. Those tickets should be used. The opportunity to hear such music must not be wasted. If she and Thomas could not go, there surely were music lovers who would grab at the chance. They must be found, quickly.

"Thomas," she said, "Call the B's and see if they would like our tickets for Saturday night—*La Traviata*—and supper afterward."

The B's were busy. She made many more phone calls that night.

My body was pain ridden, complaining. Gratefully, I accepted a sedative and turned out the light. I felt quite old and disheartened. In our twenties we don't know much about suffering. Youth and optimism go hand in hand. But in the forties and fifties there is scarcely one of us who has not lost a relative or a friend to cancer. No one is safe. I had an uneasy night.

In the morning, more talk. Besides our common love for music, we discovered similar tastes in reading. We liked each other's husband, too. What luck to have a bright and congenial roommate.

In the afternoon she went to surgery. When she had not returned after three hours I had to recognize the terrible truth.

I couldn't bear to look at Thomas's face when they finally came back to the room. The crowd of distressed friends with him, the orderlies and nurses bustling about, and the sight of Teresa's helpless body were too much for me. I should not be looking at this. I hid behind my curtain.

During the night I was awakened by her anguished cries.

"Jesus, help me," she was moaning. "What am I going to do? Help me, help me."

Was she awake? I was not sure. Sometimes people cry out in their sleep. Did she know what they had done to her?

She moaned again, now sobbing words in Italian that I couldn't understand. I had to do something.

"What can I do? Shall I call the nurse?"

She was immediately quiet. I must have wakened her. Now she was remembering. Then she said, "Yes, please, will you do that? I have so much pain."

I pressed my call button and the nurse appeared. She brought an injection for the pain, and she arranged the pillows under Teresa's arm. Quietly we lay awake. The dimly lighted room was filled with an infinite sadness.

I lived the next six days with Teresa and Thomas. The curtain between us kept them from seeing my tears when I heard them helping each other to be strong.

Oh, God, so young. The age of my firstborn. Why her and not me? I know, I know. You can't bargain with cancer.

We became dear friends. Scattered among the hours of pain and the constant physical demands, moments of revelation appeared. Each of us began to understand how strong is the will to live, and how deep are the resources of the human spirit. We saw that our griefs are universal; to become reconciled to them is our common need.

My own problems were only a nagging nuisance, as I entered Teresa's world of pain. My cancer was, the doctor told me, the best kind to have. I had called to get the results from a D & C I had in early spring.

"Doctor would like you to come and see him."

That stopped me cold. My skin prickled. What now? "May I talk with him now, please?"

"No, I'm sorry. He wants you to come to the office."

After some argument a time was set. I got up from my chair. Not a chill, but a flood of heat spread over the back of my neck. I was slightly sick in the stomach. "So that's it." I said aloud. "That's what I'm in for." I walked around from one room to another. My mind was going in all directions; I couldn't turn it off. What would it mean, to me, to all of us? I almost called back to insist on a definite statement right now. But what difference would it make? I knew what it was she wouldn't tell me.

I had to wait two days to see the doctor, so I couldn't share the knowledge that I had cancer. I told my husband that I might have bad news. Could I be wrong? But I knew I wasn't, and I spent the next two days acting my normal self, suspended between anger and fear, cursing the doctor who kept me hanging there.

After I was told that I had the best kind of cancer (lucky me), a schedule was arranged for four weeks of radiation, then a few weeks for recovery. Finally, I had the surgery that brought me to this semi-private comradeship with Teresa.

Two days after surgery the doctor told me I was cured. The tumor had been confined to the uterus. No cancer was found in the surrounding tissue. Life may go on. I'm one of the lucky ones. I am not the same, though; I know more. The edge of the shadow passed over me, too close for comfort. The long and relentless preparation gave me plenty of time to think. There is nothing like a glimpse of one's mortality to clarify the vision. I have some hallelujahs to sing. The sun on a hill and the warmth of an embrace are gifts to enjoy *now*. Love is *now*. "All things bright and beautiful" are more so.

My physiologist husband tells me something of how the brain responds to extreme crisis. The brain has a marvelous ability we use without knowing. It works like this: We are constantly choosing between alternatives, trivial and non-trivial, whenever there is a demand. It is like voting. First, we get the information, identify the problem. At once, we accept or discard certain actions. We base this choice on countless underlying attitudes, habits, and moral or ethical beliefs, all stored deep in our memories.

When a person is confronted with a real crisis, an extreme emergency, the brain displays its greatest power. The network of signals is tuned at once to responding to its immense task. What to do? Like turning on your television, you tune first to get the right channel, then the color, the light or dark, the intensity of the picture. We use both sides of the brain; one side leaps to decision, the other side, with its ability to compare, moderates and re-enforces. This interaction helps one achieve a sense of direction. Trivial aspects are discarded unconsciously. We are able to see the realities of the situation.

Then the sources of strength within us rise to save us. These were trained into us in the past. They are so deep we don't know where we got them. We may receive courage learned at a mother's knee, or values for conduct born out of friendship, or the faith and optimism of religious belief. These treasures, deep in the vaults of memory, come to our rescue when we let them. It is clear that we can depend on our minds and bodies far more than we have ever imagined.

I watched with astonishment this renewing process going on in my roommate. When the report was bad, she died a little. Then the underlying strengths within her began to take over. She faced the truth. Then she started planning what to do about it.

More treatment was necessary. Teresa's first concern was the security of her little Licia. Thomas was wonderful; she could rely on his gentle strength. But he could not do everything; help was needed.

"I know my mother will want to come," she said. "I need her here, but I can't tell her about the mastectomy."

"You have to tell her."

"Yes, I'll tell her, but not on the telephone. I can't do that. She would be so upset. She could have a heart attack right on the phone. And to travel with that on her mind—it would be terrible for her. No, I must tell her something to get her to come, then I can be with her to break the bad news."

I agreed that such news was better divulged in person.

"You help me think of something, Pat," she continued. "What would make me come to the hospital, but not be too serious…? Maybe I could say I have peritonitis, what do you think?"

"Oh, I don't think so," I said quickly. "That would be rather unusual. She might wonder about that. Surely, there's a more simple ailment…"

Finally we decided on a D & C.

"That will be reasonable," said Teresa. "She had that a couple of times herself. She won't worry too much about that. I'll call her."

Her mother spoke only Italian.

The conversation began with a cheery, "Ciao, Mama." After that a flood of animated Italian poured forth, with frequent pauses, interruptions, and ardent persuasions. At last, I heard her say, "Okay, I'll see you, Mama," and she hung up, laughing and crying helplessly.

"Oh, what a mess I got into! Poor Mama. She couldn't understand why I need help if I only had a D & C. She said, 'It's nothing. I had it three times; you'll never notice it.' Then I told her I was a little bit pregnant and had a miscarriage, and she scolded me for not being careful! I kept getting in deeper. It was so hilarious!"

Both of us were holding our stitches. "At last," Teresa continued, "I managed to convince her. She will come. Thomas can meet her and bring her here. Then she will know." Tears came again as she pictured her mother's grief.

The next day a psychologist came in to talk with Teresa. She was loaded with ideas about coping with the problems of adjustment. She wanted to help Teresa learn how to accept her loss. She looked bewildered when she left. There was no bitterness in Teresa. She was not crying, "Why me?" She didn't consider that she had been unfairly singled out for tragedy. She understood that we all are vulnerable.

"That was so funny," she told me. "She thought I would blame somebody. How can I blame? Everybody has trouble."

She knew how to be quiet and let the healing enter.

Though we were novices we knew a lot about cancer. We talked about the problems of our bodies, and problems, too, with other people. We had no patience with a cover up; we had to be honest. Neither of us could abide the cheerful visitors who said idiotically, "You'll be fine." What did they know? Neither did we admire those who evaded the issue altogether. It was an insult to pretend that nothing was wrong.

I admit that at first I had trouble saying, "I have cancer."

How uncomfortable for the other person. Better to say, "The thing the doctor called a polyp turned out to be malignant." But malignant is not a nice word either; "cancer" and "malignant" are both ugly. There is no pleasant word to dispel the scent of danger. After a few tries I learned to say, "I feel all right, but I do have a problem. I'm having treatment for cancer of the uterus." But you can't stop there. It's a good idea to give your listener a few casual details to allow her time to recover.

For days after surgery Teresa suffered agonizing pain. The nurses were gentle and sympathetic, with the exception of one brawny blond whose bosom jutted like a mansard roof beneath her determined chin. Without ceremony she would haul Teresa up in the bed and deposit her in position like a sack of grain. Thomas called her Brunhilda. We tried to steer clear of her.

The healing began. At first we both walked slightly bent, with one arm across the front of the body, old women protecting our wounds. The stitches hurt when we laughed at each other.

Thomas laughed with Teresa, too. With a conjurer's flourish, he presented to her a gift of black sweet cherries. She told me about a beautiful day they had spent in the orchards, climbing the trees, soaking up the smells and the color, picking and eating in the hot sun. Comfort me with cherries.

Teresa didn't like chrysanthemums. In Italy they are funeral flowers. Pleading lack of space, I sent mine home.

Pretty nightgowns and robes were out. I had to change often because of constant drenching sweats. Teresa had a more visible problem. Fluids oozed though the extensive bandages on her side and stained her gown and bed linen, so that she often felt unkempt. It's hard to pretty up cancer.

We went about comfortably in the ubiquitous short hospital gowns, tied at the back of the neck, and changed a couple of times a day. Teresa's gown was often flapping open because she couldn't manage the ties. I could see her beautiful suntanned back with only a small light triangle where her bikini had been. Thomas gave a wolfish whistle when she turned her back on him.

The young nurses became our good friends and ran in often when they had a few free minutes. Teresa gave the last two opera tickets to one of them. We had a lively discussion about what she should wear to the gala matinee.

These were sunny moments when life was simple, when we put sorrow away in a corner behind the door.

In this book, Teresa describes her own emotions when breast cancer invaded her body. She writes of mourning; fear and pain are her companions. She speaks with intensity of the quality of life. She has no magic formula for dealing with cancer. But she has thought and learned a great deal about it, and what she has gleaned is presented here. In sharing her experiences, she shares her discoveries, and her methods for handling that old devil, doubt. She opens her treasure house for us.

Her writing is both poetic and practical. This is also her way of life. She loves, works, enjoys, and is eternally vigilant.

I have had half a dozen roommates during several hospital stays. Some of these women were pleasant; some were boring; most faded into a clouded "other time." Not so,

Teresa. If I never saw her again, I would still be blessed by her valiant and loving spirit. The gifts that we unwrapped during that week together are safely tucked away in the support system of my memory. Take one or more as needed.

Pat Wolterink
1972

Preface

I wrote this book because, as a young mother who experienced breast cancer, I searched for a book like this and found nothing. All the available non-technical writings seemed aimed at the middle-aged woman whose children were teenagers or adults.

I hope to reach the young female relatives of breast cancer patients, for statistics show that these young women are at much higher risk of contracting the disease than other women. In the *New York Times* (November 17, 1976), an article entitled "Breast Cancer: Ways of Telling a High Risk" by Jane E. Brody mentions many factors involved. For example, the author says, "On the average, close blood relatives of breast cancer patients, their daughters, sisters, maternal aunts and nieces—are two to three times more likely to get breast cancer than women whose families are free of the disease." Also, "If the cancer was bilateral (in both breasts) and also occurred before the woman had reached menopause, the risk to her relatives was nine times higher than expected—giving them a nearly 50 percent chance of developing breast cancer."

If only one person can be helped, my book will have served its purpose.

I am also eager to comfort and help those women who have already been told that they have cancer. No book, no words can ever entirely remove the dread and anguish from their hearts, but I hope this will help allay their fears and give them hope.

Very often in a health crisis, the children, spouse, friends, and relatives of the patient are thrown on their own resources—abandoned and alone in their sadness. This book speaks to those loved persons surrounding the breast cancer patient; people who want to help and feel so totally helpless. I want women to learn how to let their children, even very young ones, give them comfort. A young child has a powerful, positive effect on the morale of a seriously ill person. We can't pretend to be the "omnipotent" adult when the surgeon tells us we are in mortal danger.

The husband and parents of a breast cancer patient need to know what changes will occur in the family after surgery. It is not easy to live day by day. The patient, family, and friends find themselves oscillating from the heights to the depths; neither is it easy for the members of the family to live with a woman who has the psychology of a survivor, for whom every moment counts.

If the patient, her family, and her friends can work together as a group to share all aspects of cancer—the discovery of the disease, diagnosis, treatment, recovery, and a return to normal living—the problems can be approached sympathetically and compassionately. Then cancer can be dealt with more effectively. As Franklin Delano Roosevelt said, "We have nothing to fear but fear itself." It is fear and isolation which destroy the spirit, and love can conquer fear.

I was born in Capistrano, a small town in southern Italy, in 1942, in the midst of World War II. At the time of my birth, our town was miraculously spared from enemy bombing. To celebrate the occasion, my dearest Aunt Maria, a nun who had just arrived from her bombed convent, called the neighboring ladies and made my first little dress from the only piece of cloth lying around, an Italian flag.

I spent my first three years near Serra San Bruno, a beautiful part of the country with a majestic monastery covered by lovely pines. These pines used to give me shelter from sudden rain when I, so oblivious to everything, was involved in childhood play. Many years later, the pines near a monastery, this time in Michigan, provided a metaphor for my long process of healing and acceptance.

My older sister, who used to take care of me and make sure I did not accept chocolates from liberating soldiers, tells me that I loved to listen to the American troops speaking English. One day, softened by my admiration for these young men, she let me accept a chocolate from one of them. Worse still, she let me eat the chocolate, thus breaking one of my father's strict rules—not to accept anything from strangers.

War in Italy was a time of horror. As I grew up in the postwar reconstruction period, our environment was completely polluted and destroyed by the war. I very early witnessed the ugliness of war when my playmate was seriously injured by the explosion of a "cute" little box we had found nearby.

Yet, in spite of poverty, famine, and the prolonged suffering, people knew how to welcome joyous moments: the feast of a Madonna, a marching band, a visiting opera company, a theater group, a wedding. We had so little, yet so much! We were free from material possessions, for money had no buying power. One day my grandfather actually used it as toilet paper.

To flee from postwar depression (for we lost everything during the war), my father and my two eldest sisters immigrated to Canada, and my mother and I later joined them. My fourth sister married an Australian, and she too left our beloved Italy.

My journey to Canada, a country I would later come to love, was painful, for at the age of 17 it is difficult to leave one's milieu, no matter how hard life is. How I cried as we drove away from the little town where I had learned so much of vital importance to me. I missed the disabled man in our town whose knowledge of opera surpassed that of any opera singer, and who knew by heart every note both vocally and instrumentally. How angry he would grow when I did not pay attention to his anvil chorus or Aida's judgment. I loved his visiting our house every night after supper to entertain and enlighten us. I can still hear the solemn knock at the door; not the timid tap of an intruder but the strong knock of a performer.

In contrast to these happy memories, Canada at first seemed like a battleground. I wanted to continue my education, yet I had no knowledge of English. At my father's urging, I went to school every day at the age of 19 surrounded by 14-year-olds in the ninth grade.

It was painful; yet, I knew I had to overcome the language barrier. How wonderful it would be to read Shakespeare in English—I, who had to memorize *Hamlet* in my high school in Italy. I was very excited to read English works in the original. Bernard Shaw had always been one of my favorites. I became so intoxicated with his writings that I stopped taking my afternoon siesta in the last desk of the classroom and from then on my progress flourished.

In no time, I penetrated the great country of Canada, where I taught English as a second language for several years and became a proud citizen. However, my difficulties with a new environment were not yet over.

While 1968 began with joy when I married a young, brilliant American lawyer named Thomas Carlson, our honeymoon was abruptly terminated by the army. We were sent to Fort Knox, Kentucky, where once more I witnessed the agony of war, this time as an older and more painfully aware person. I became an English teacher at the Army Education Center, where every day I met with three classes of young soldiers preparing for their high school equivalency diploma, many of whom had spent time in Vietnam and were full of horror stories. How often I sobbed with those boys— those who were lucky enough to return brought back to me the atrocity of another war.

Yet, all through this time my home life with Thomas matured into a beautiful blend of my own inborn Italian exuberance and his calm, meditative Scandinavian personality.

We were blessed with the birth of a magnificent child, who would later give me the strength to move mountains, to stand unbearable pain; I, who, according to my sister Nina, used to faint at the sight of blood.

My sisters and my mother, though far away, shared with me my innermost suffering, for we were all so close in spirit. We could always sense when one of us was in pain. As my sister Gina said, "Why did it have to happen to you, and not to me instead?" In Italy we were one body, all seven of us, and thanks to that cohesive force which enveloped us night and day in our one-room war refuge, in our family gatherings at night in front of the fireplace, on the terrace sunbathing, we overcame any separation. There is a bond between us that not even death can destroy.

To complete the Carlson family, there lives a proud, 94-year-old grandmother, whose background is not dissimilar to mine. She, too, left her native land, Sweden, when she was a teenager.

There seems to be nothing new in this world, just a creative force which crosses oceans only to manifest itself in a different language. Whether from Italy, Sweden, Canada, or anywhere else, like the pines we are universal beings, for we speak of living, an art common to all.

Teresa Carlson
1976

PART I: VIA DOLOROSA

1

The First Fall

The sun shines, the sky is clear, and a gentle zephyr wafts the many scents of summer. Yet just out of sight, behind a cloud, can hide a potential storm. And in a blink, the breeze becomes a hurricane. Still, we continue to enjoy the summer bliss as if we were in absolute control of our world and our lives. Until, for many of us, the tempest comes and our strength and vision are called to task.

The tempest that caught me unawares is cancer. Its initial signs are for some the last call; for others, the beginning of a struggle where the hope of victory is slim. Though the fight at times becomes overwhelming, and the storm threatens total destruction, we push on, because the instinct to survive is intrinsic and spontaneous.

November 1971 marked the beginning of my *via dolorosa*—my path of sorrow. I was 29 years old. It started one Sunday afternoon. I woke from a nap, and had dreamt that I had a lump in my right breast. I was too terrified to check it immediately. But the dream was a reality. The lump was there.

The following day, my husband, our one-year-old baby and I went to the gynecologist, who, to my surprise, thought nothing of it. He said it was nothing to worry about. At worst, it was a swollen milk gland. He asked the nurse to show me a short movie about breast examination and bade me goodbye until the following year. I sat through the film wondering why I needed to watch it. I had already discovered a lump. Obviously, I knew how to examine myself. I was thoroughly confused, but relieved that the doctor wasn't concerned. On the way home, I thought briefly about getting a second opinion, but it never materialized.

Five months later, in April 1972, having indulged in too much early spring sunbathing, I caught a severe cold which brought me to the doctor; this time, a general practitioner. As I was leaving his office, a booklet prominently displayed on the receptionist's desk caught my eye. I picked it up, opened it hastily and read, "If you have a lump in your breast, don't walk but run to the doctor." I did exactly that. I ran back into the doctor's office, rudely interrupting an examination. I showed him the lump, and he immediately had the nurse check me into the hospital the next day for a biopsy. Tears streaming down my face, I raced outside to inform my husband who was cheerfully enjoying our 17-month-old daughter, Licia. I wished I could join in their laughter. Instead, my tears drowned it.

We returned to the gynecologist ("Dr. X"), who, this

time, was alarmed to find the lump there. I could not believe my ears. The same lump, that five months ago did not move him, was suddenly a source of concern. Strange, I thought. I would later learn that Dr. X suffered from narcolepsy, an illness characterized by brief attacks of deep sleep—this came as no surprise.

The following day, we consulted a surgeon, Dr. Harold Schmidt, who saw no reason for alarm, as there were no apparent cancer signs. The earliest I could be admitted into the hospital was in a week. Even though the surgeon was reassuring, I had a premonition that my situation was far from good.

The week that followed was agonizing. Major decisions had to be made. Dr. Schmidt had explained his method of dealing with the lump, and told us we were free to consult with or choose another surgeon who espoused a different philosophy.

I initially preferred to begin with just the biopsy, and later decide on any further surgery. But Dr. Schmidt convinced me that the chance of successful surgery was greater if performed immediately. He believed, for biopsy purposes, in the freezing of a section, whereby the lump and several other samples of breast tissue would be rushed for examination by a pathologist. The patient at that stage would already be under general anesthesia, so that if the lump were malignant, the surgeon would then proceed with a radical mastectomy—the removal of the breast, along with its underlying muscles and the lymph glands that drain it. The smaller the lump, the more effective the surgery, and the better the odds of survival. He also felt that the removal of the lymph nodes was essential to ascertain the extent of the cancer, and to determine post-surgical methods of treatment such as chemotherapy, radiation, or both.

Feeling confident in his ability as a surgeon and secure under his care, I signed the paper. I respected his integrity and his skill, and was very touched by his sensitivity to my situation.

In spite of all the reassurance I received from my husband and friends, I was worried. Somehow, I knew it was malignant. Everyone said that it was obviously nothing; most women have lumps some time or other in their lives. I had nothing to worry about; I was the picture of health.

I wished that even one person would say, "What if it *is* malignant, then what...?" and invite me to open my Pandora's box, already packed with fears, confusion, and certainty of a loss that would affect not only my physical and emotional state, but shake the foundations of my concept of womanhood. But no one asked, so I suffered in lonely silence, preparing for battle like a good soldier.

I spent many hours mourning the anticipated loss of a breast and days at the library reading about cancer and its implications. An article in *Time* magazine offered me some comfort. On the cover of that week's issue was a picture of a young girl who had had breast reconstruction. She was wearing a bikini. That image flashed in front of my eyes as I continued the private mourning in the depths of my being.

I soon discovered that my fears surrounding the loss of a breast transcended the loss of sex appeal. My suffering was twofold. As an attractive young woman, perhaps influenced by the American obsession with sexiness, I considered the breasts aesthetically essential. I loved to wear bikinis, décolleté dresses, braless dresses, and I felt great in them. Yet, a much stronger fear seized me. My "Italianness" was being threatened.

As an Italian, I viewed the breast not as a sexual attribute, but as a life-sustaining organ. How many women had I seen in southern Italy, infant at their breast, giving of themselves both in spirit and in body? I still see them washing at the fountain before nursing, to refresh their tired bodies and to prepare for this blessed act after a hard day's work in the fields. How could I forget the countless times I went to call the wet nurse when my little cousin was ready to be fed? How could I then conceive of such a loss?

My whole concept of motherhood was at stake—a concept well shaped by Renaissance art, by all the beautiful Madonnas cradling infant at breast. A sublime picture! I loved to evoke them all, but especially one painting by Leonardo da Vinci: Madonna Litta, sitting in absolute peace, her baby at her breast. What harmony I found in the recollection; what discord in my reality.

For me it was inconceivable to be deprived of a breast for nursing my future child; the child I was hoping to conceive soon. I wanted more children. I wanted to give myself wholly to future offspring as I did with Licia, and as my mother did me. How insignificant the loss of sexiness seemed in comparison. I realized that I was immersed in the deep waters of life, not wading the shallow waters of appearances.

This notion of Madonna motherhood overpowered me, and obscured the more serious threat that cancer brings—the loss of life. I read about it but couldn't quite accept it. I felt like the soldiers in Tolstoy's *War and Peace* who, on their way to battle, stopped to pet dogs, to play with them, to laugh and enjoy the moment. How wonderful that we possess such a safety valve—a valve that shuts out pieces of reality so we can slowly and systematically suffer each small part of a loss without being overwhelmed by the totality of it.

Death never entered my mind. Perhaps such a thought would have crushed me entirely, for I was still an infant in the world of suffering. How marvelously organized our body is; how well equipped we are. We perceive only what we can digest; only what we can carry without collapsing under the weight. As the Christian maxim teaches, no cross is too heavy to bear. This became so clear to me.

The night in the hospital before surgery was the nadir of my anguish. The overarching fear of losing a breast was now compounded by other worries—the anesthetic, the actual surgery, the pain. Would I be able to withstand such intense pain—I, who had never suffered any serious physical pain, except in childbirth? But that was the pain of creating, not of loss.

My fears were not allayed by my roommate, who was lying in bed motionless, moaning faintly. I went to her, touched her forehead, and cried, for I knew that tomorrow I would be moaning too, only maybe a little louder. I stood there watching this beautiful woman who was later to become a good friend. I looked long and deep into my new mirror, and I cried.

My reverie was broken by the cheerful voice of the nurse, asking me to undress and put on the hospital gown. I was still in my summer outfit. I felt so healthy in it, so vibrant. In the hospital gown, I felt helpless. Once in bed, the series of preoperative tests began. I had become a patient. It is amazing how quickly one shifts from a regular person to the dehumanized anonymity of a patient. "I adapt beautifully," I thought.

I could not fall asleep that night. I thought of my little girl finding herself suddenly without her mother. I wished she had come along with us when I checked in. Instead, I left her sleeping. Poor little baby, what will she think of me? Why didn't I tell her I would be back soon? I began to miss her terribly. I felt so confused; I didn't know what to do. Should I call home and talk to her? How can a 17-month-old infant understand my anguish? I didn't even know if I would be able to speak; I felt a big lump in my throat.

Suddenly, I was a child again myself. I remembered my home in Italy and how we all prayed together in times of crisis. I knelt down and began to say the Lord's Prayer. After the words, "Thy will be done," I could continue no longer. I felt so ethereal and so peaceful that I fell asleep. I fell asleep in God's hands and woke to the gentle touch of my husband's hand the following morning.

Six hours later, I woke from the artificial sleep of anesthesia, only this time to the knowledge that the lump was malignant and that I had had a radical mastectomy. This came as no shock to me. Dr. Schmidt, the surgeon, had whispered it to me several times in the recovery room. And my husband's eyes communicated it all.

But I had already lived the loss so intensively that it was now old hat. I was ready to begin the work of healing. My husband reassured me that together we could overcome any obstacles. I felt very much at peace. My main task was now to heal fast. Every ounce of strength I had left was to be geared toward mending. I could not burden my mind with thoughts of "Why me?" or attachment to anger. I had to dispel any anxiety from my mind so that the body could do its work unimpaired.

The surgeon marveled at how peaceful I looked the following day and explained the importance of remaining calm and resting so the body can mobilize all its forces toward healing. That made sense to me. Poor body, how could it cope with mental anguish when it had so much mending to do? I also felt relieved that I was not suffering alone any longer. I could share every pain with my Thomas and together manage beautifully. Even physical pain became shareable.

For the five days that followed, we were calm and happy in our confidence that life would soon be as beautiful as before, and perhaps even a little fuller. Licia came to see me. How quiet and reserved she was. She, too, had been wounded. Her first words were, "Mommy, *preghiamo Padre Nostro*." She wanted me to say the "Our Father" with her. She joined her little hands in prayer. What a joy! As young as she was, she too found refuge in the Lord's Prayer. What a strange coincidence that the same prayer that lulled me to sleep before surgery was the one Licia wanted to say just then.

I longed to hold her, but I couldn't. Cast-like bandages covered my whole breast area, and the arm on the operated side was immobile. To make the slightest movement was excruciating. But her presence alone was healing, her smile contagious; her eyes shone with the promise of life. Her five-minute visits were reinvigorating. With her I did not have to explain how I felt; holding hands was enough.

How powerful small children are! I wished America's generations were not so isolated; that old and sick people were in closer contact with the young and healthy, to be rejuvenated by them. I longed for a moment to live in Italy, where the old and the young were not miles apart but a footstep away. I resolved right then to take Licia to retirement homes and share her with them. My grandfather used to say that as long as there were children around, one never felt old. I understood perfectly what he meant for I, too, was experiencing the simple but mighty healing power of a child.

The three of us loved our five minutes together, all sitting cozily on the hospital bed. I was healing splendidly. There was no need for skin grafting. All seemed well again. And we were now looking forward to our future together, assured that this was no more than a small black cloud in the sky.

But this peaceful existence was soon to end, for it was only the calm eye of the hurricane. Before long, we would again be caught in its whirlwind.

2

Recovery

*Which one of us can listen to the hymn of the
brook, while the tempest roars.*

Kahlil Gibran

The pathologist's report came back and two-thirds of the
lymph nodes were cancerous. This was serious. The surgeon
voiced his fears honestly and as gently as he could. "Things
are not as good as we thought," he said. Unsure how grave
my case was, he tried to explain it statistically: "If there were
100 women in your situation, 75 would survive a year, 25
would not, and I don't know where to put you."

Goodbye dreams of a peaceful tomorrow. Goodbye
laughter! A dreadful shadow darkened our world. We felt it
but we did not speak of it. I suppose it had been there all
along, looming, but we had not recognized it or even
acknowledged it. Like a night visitor dressed in black, it had

passed unnoticed. But now, we felt its presence, and it seemed more powerful than all our previous fears. Death, with all its brutality, crept into our hearts. We were now suspended between life and death. Language ceased; a tear, a squeezing of a hand was all we could express.

For a cancer patient, surgery is unfortunately only the first step. Then a long road begins: tests, radiation, chemotherapy, all or some combination of these. However, it is through this laborious road that one begins to reach a different plateau of life. I felt like Dante in *The Inferno*, walking on a dark road in the woods. I did not know where I was going, but with Thomas and Licia, I would be able to cross even the River Styx. Like Dante, I needed a guide, a Virgil, to help me through this terrestrial hell, and a Beatrice to show me the new vision of life.

My Virgil was my husband, who constantly stood by my side and helped me through every bandage change and saw to it that I was treated with the utmost gentleness. A bandage change would not normally be such an ordeal, but after a few days of rebandaging the wound, I developed tape burns. Ripping the tape off abruptly caused excruciating pain. For the first few times, Thomas held my hand and attempted to amuse me with his wonderful humor, but as the pain became more intolerable, he tactfully volunteered to take over. He had a marvelous technique: with one hand he lifted a corner of the tape, and with the other he held down the skin to minimize the pulling. He performed this procedure so slowly and so gently that I hardly felt any pain. Once the wound was exposed, the nurse took over.

This was a good experience for both of us. It gave

Thomas a chance to view the wound and begin adjusting to the way my body looked. It also afforded him the opportunity to give me reassuring reports about the condition of the wound.

The first time he saw it must have been a shocking experience. However, his face disclosed no horror. Instead, he exclaimed encouragingly: "Dr. Schmidt is an artist; he did a beautiful job. It looks really good." What an actor he was! Later, he told me that he was shocked.

"The shock came because of its nature as a wound, and not its location. I would have felt the same had you had a bad burn on the leg or the arm. The fact that a breast had been removed didn't seem to have much relevance. In fact, there is nothing pretty about any kind of wound, but that is something that only time heals, both physically and psychologically."

He also said that the first time he pulled the bandages off, he felt a numbing effect. The wound looked bad, but he wasn't going to tell me that. He held his breath and did his job. After four or five times, it became routine.

He read to me to lull the pain and soothe me during the long evenings. At night, we are closer to thoughts of death. The sense of desolation can be overpowering if one is alone in a hospital room. The somber lights, the whispering, the wilting flowers, and the quiet one must maintain. I was grateful that visiting regulations were relaxed so that Thomas could stay with me until I fell asleep. I found it very comforting to close my eyes holding his hand and feeling the flow of life between us.

My Beatrice was my little Licia, an 18-month-old who gave me the strength to move mountains. How quiet she was,

14

how spiritual. She led me into prayer. As young as she was, she found refuge in the Lord. This gave me comfort, for if I were to die, at least I had instilled in her the concept of God. Each time I held her fragile, supportive hand, I experienced the ecstasy of life. My Beatrice was giving me a vision of Heaven even though she reproached me repeatedly for having temporarily disappeared from her life.

My return home was slightly overshadowed by the prospect of having radiation therapy. I had read about the effect of radiation on healthy cells and the possible damage to the lungs. However, this apprehension was short-lived. The surgeon was unsure at this point whether radiation would even be effective. A bone scan would have to be done to determine whether the cancer had become systemic; that is, whether it had penetrated into the bone marrow.

We were now to face a new fear. Oh, how I wished and hoped and prayed that the bone scan would be negative, so I could have the localized radiation on the sternum (breast bone). What seemed an ordeal a short while ago was now the very thing for which I was praying. How relative our fears are! I recalled the adage I once saw on a bumper sticker: "I cried because I had no shoes, until I saw a man who had no feet!"

Despite the emotional confusion, I was exhilarated at the thought of going home. I longed for that familiar setting: my little girl's room, the crib by which I had stood so many nights singing her lullabies.

The homecoming was splendid. Thomas and my mother prepared our home as if a visitor from another country were to arrive. Everything was beautifully arranged. The bed was made in the Italian style, with embroidered linen and a satin bedspread fit for a queen; a bottle of champagne was on the table. Home, however, was not complete without Licia, who was on her way from Grandmother Carlson's house. My neck stiffened looking out the window for Grandfather's car. When Licia finally arrived, she saw me; but instead of holding onto me, she ran around the house like a little bird who, after a long search, has at last found its home, and has to make sure it is the right home. We were all excited. We drank champagne as if it were the nectar of normality and love.

When Licia went to bed that night, I wanted to be near her to sing our favorite songs. How feeble I was! I knelt down to gather my strength, and Licia, thinking I wanted to pray, began to sing the "Our Father."

Now that I was home, I became so conscious of strength. At the hospital, everyone was so weak that each patient mirrored the other. The slow walks down the corridor were a great accomplishment. At home, however, it was a different story. The healthy members of the family were the standard. At home, one's weakness is in sharp contrast to the buzzing around of the fit. It is, in a way, a temptation that one must acknowledge and learn to overcome. It is like looking at yourself in a magnifying glass. Everything becomes huge.

I soon realized that returning from the helplessness of being a patient to a normal condition of healthy independence is more difficult than the reverse. I recalled what a short transition it was for me to become a patient 12 days ago. I realized this second adjustment was much harder, and I owed it to myself and to my family to manage it with as little stress as possible. A favorite saying of Gestalt followers is, "Do not push the river." I knew I could not push myself back into life, but would have to surrender to the tide.

I decided I was going to treat myself firmly, but gently. I was going to give myself time to heal, to recover my strength, and to accept help. A disabled skier does not place himself at the top of a hill and plunge down. So why should I set unattainable goals? I had undergone tremendous stress and suffering during the past month. Why add more? To live each day became my goal. To think in terms of one day at a time was my plan.

As I knew that my first week at home would be quite an adjustment, I kept a very simple schedule. My goals were not overly ambitious, and could be easily met. Too often, I feel, we set unrealistic goals, and when we fail to achieve them, we become frustrated and depressed. Life throws at us enough discouraging experiences; I was not looking to add my own. I was extremely careful not to allow myself to fall into depression.

My primary concern was restoring the mobility of my arm. Radical mastectomy involves the removal of the pectoral muscles. Thus, a new set of muscles on the inner arm between the shoulder and elbow has to be trained to do the work previously done by the pectoral muscles. A series of exercises must be performed daily in order to get the arm functional again. The exercises were painful and I admit I did not look forward to them.

Licia loved to mark on the wall how far I could lift my arm. She enjoyed the role of parent-teacher. We would both face the wall and with our hands, climb the wall as far as we could. Licia insisted that every millimeter—even the slightest progress—was recorded. (A small consolation for the mastectomy patient is that she will never have hanging underarms as she ages, if she is lucky enough to reach old age.)

The exercises consumed a lot of energy and time, as I had to do them regularly, three times a day. After each session, Licia and I would be rewarded with a bowl of fresh fruits, beautifully arranged by my mother, who now and then would shed a tender tear as she watched our efforts. Afterward, we would take a short rest to regain strength for a brief walk, or to read a story to my little helper.

As the exercises were exhausting, I was careful not to overexert myself with too many other activities. I made sure to save my energies for the exercises, as I was determined to get the arm back in shape so that I could lift Licia up and hug her as before. Dr. Schmidt explained that this was critical to do in the two weeks following my return home, because otherwise, the arm would atrophy and I would never regain full control. The specter of such a possibility motivated me to stick with the harsh routine.

In this way, my first two weeks at home were spent doing very little, by normal standards, but a great deal for someone who has undergone major surgery. Even sitting at the table and eating was a challenge after two weeks in a hospital bed. I found outings, other than simple walks, very tiring. I avoided shopping centers and large crowds.

In the evenings, after Licia went to bed, I always managed to spend some time with Thomas. For that, too, I had to conserve energy. I made sure that I had a nap before he came home so that I did not look or feel drained. I found those quiet moments very beautiful. In a way, we were learning to be together again. Being home can be wearing; however, if you preserve your resources it can be quite a healing experience. The key is to live simply and prudently, and above all, to take one day at a time.

The bone scan was scheduled for Friday. The suspense was unbearable. We had to wait all weekend for the results. The loss of my breast was fading into the past. We never talked about it; there was so much more to think and worry about.

My little Beatrice, however, gave me glimpses of joy and heaven. She commanded that I participate in the many calls of life even though the shadow of death hovered over me. What a bother death is when one has little children to care for. Children are powerful! They can dispel the night with their bold demands, with their quaint humor, and with their quiet wisdom.

By Sunday, Licia had me so involved in her activities and her routines that at times nothing seemed to have changed. Cancer was far away; life was calling me to partake of its many rituals and blessings. Licia and I played, read books, sang songs, but mostly, we did the exercises.

When I could finally raise my arm completely over my head, we were all excited and Licia clapped her hands in delight. She was suspended between this joy and her puzzlement over such a celebration for a simple thing like raising your arms. Her understandable confusion revealed the poignancy of my experience. We take for granted the smooth functioning of our bodies. I felt like an alpinist, proud but exhausted. My husband gave me a tennis racket as a present, and Licia and I would go outside and bang the ball against the back of the school building. Licia, young as she was, felt proud and somewhat responsible for my accomplishments.

I realized during this ordeal that it is important to involve children in our struggles. Yet, we must be mindful not to drown the child under their weight. Children are wise; if left alone, they tend to absorb as much as they can handle. If they are overwhelmed by the totality of a problem, however, they will break. We must not belabor our suffering; rather, we should learn from them to respond to this beautiful mechanism we have within which helps us survive tragedies. It takes great geniuses like Tolstoy to discover the mind's power to obstruct all of reality, so that survival is ensured. But it takes children to show us how to use such power. Children select and reject, intuitively, each aspect of a problem, and deal with it gradually as they develop strength.

The bone scan was negative; there was no trace of cancer in the bones. Once I had sufficiently healed, I began radiation treatment. The first session was traumatic. For the first time since surgery, I lost my patience, and resented terribly being treated together with older people. I felt I did not belong there.

The sight of the radiation therapy room frightened me—a huge machine hung down with a gurney under it. I had no idea how close the machine was going to come to me and, alone in that dismal room, I felt crushed, and for the first time, angry. But the anger did not last long. I was about to be reminded again of the relativity of suffering.

When I came out of the radiation room, I saw my husband holding a little baby while the mother went to the ladies' room. The infant was only six months old and was the next patient to enter the dismal room. I regretted my anger and my words, "God, I do not belong here." If that little child could speak, he would have had the right to say, "What am I doing here with this old Teresa Carlson?" I was once again very much humbled, and from then on, I began to think about the universality of suffering. I decided that anger is not constructive, and I began to think very positively about the manner of my living.

For the following four weeks, I faced that gloomy room every morning at eight. To calm myself, as soon as I lay down on the gurney, I did abdominal breathing exercises. I was conscious of the fact that those dangerous rays were also killing healthy cells in me. To dispel that horrible thought, I deliberately directed my mind to a joyful memory. One morning I recalled how vibrant I was during my pregnancy, how I felt the first sign of life. I burst into laughter as I recalled when, in my last week of pregnancy, a major kick from Licia lifted up my dress. I was writing a political science examination at the time. The look on the professor's face was something to behold. He could easily handle any political philosophy controversy, but a birth? No, thank you! With those pictures flashing through my mind, I was able to reconcile to that dismal room.

Since radiation therapy was exhausting, I found I needed a lot of rest as soon as I got home. I felt tired and nauseous most of the time. The last two weeks of the therapy presented another problem. I was unable to swallow; it was as though a lump were lodged in my throat. This, I found, was a very dangerous period in terms of physical and mental health. It seemed so easy to succumb to the horror of cancer. However, to prevent myself from getting weak, I ate very well and abundantly during the first two weeks of treatment. When the symptoms worsened, I continued eating well, painful though it was. I took in plenty of liquids and soft foods whether my stomach retained them or not.

I found the advice the captain of the ship gave me when I immigrated to Canada in 1958 particularly helpful. "Never stop coming to the dining room," he said, "whether you feel nauseous or not. Better to throw up food than bile." I was not sure about his logic then, but I followed his advice, and to my surprise, it did work. I was one of the few people who walked off the ship without needing help when we landed in Halifax. Likewise, I survived the radiation without too much physical strain or mental anguish. It is extremely important to keep strong, and to recognize radiation therapy as a temporary inconvenience.

I also kept myself cheerful with light reading; nothing too serious or heavy. When I was not resting, I treated myself to the simple pleasures of life, like healthy walks, sunsets, children's songs, and good company. I surrounded myself with people who had a cheerful disposition, rather than those who pitied me constantly. Most of all, I avoided conflicts. I had wonderful help from my mother and my mother-in-law, who ran the household. I contributed by doing a light job every day. By the time the radiation therapy was over, I was able to do more and more and slowly take over the household duties.

For the woman who has neither a mother nor a mother-in-law willing and able to help, specific jobs can be delegated to the husband, the children, and to loving neighbors. If this is not possible and hired assistance is not feasible, there are many church organizations made up of wonderful men and women who will help with the children, the cooking, and the rest. Do not try to be heroic and overexert yourself. The strength of this country is evidenced in its voluntary task force. Don't be shy to accept the help. You may give immense pleasure to someone who is happy to feel useful and share your burden.

Soon I would have to face other terrible aspects of my illness.

After radiation, both the radiologist and the surgeon advised me against having any more children. What a blow that was! I had wanted more children. Not only for me, but for my little girl. I wanted her to enjoy an exciting family as I had, surrounded by four sisters. I understood the reasoning behind the advice. Research indicates the danger of bearing children following radiation, due to the possibility of dormant cancerous cells floating through the body, which can be activated by pregnancy. Radiation may also cause deformed children. I understood; yet, I was intensely disappointed.

Still another disappointment awaited me. I learned that I could not have breast reconstruction like the girl in *Time* magazine. With a radical mastectomy, reconstruction was impossible, as there was nothing left to build upon. Yet, this disappointment, juxtaposed to my inability to have more children, became less significant. Again, my maternal instinct eclipsed the cosmetic concern.

This was a debilitating period. That Sunday, we went to

church, and the thought gently settled in my mind, slowly soothing my broken spirit. "Should a man nurse his anger against his fellows and expect healing from the Lord?" This stayed with me all day. I thought how well I had recovered from surgery, how strong my arm was becoming, how peaceful I felt now that I had experienced and survived my losses. I felt no anger for Dr. X, who had originally misdiagnosed me; rather, I felt sorry for him, and worried about the effects his illness may have on others.

I was very much in a contemplative mood. I cherished and enjoyed this time of inactivity. I felt like the child who needs so much sleep for the brain to sort out all the stimuli that bombard him daily. To renew my spirit, I had to sit back and let life find me. There were no immediate calls for activity, and for this I was thankful. Yet, was I cured? I should have been weighed down by such a question, but I let it pass by like a cloud on a spring day.

I was very gentle with myself and tried to recall only happy events, so as not to disturb the mental healing that was taking place. I felt joyful for all I had known—Thomas's love, Licia's cheer, my parents' total devotion. When love is known in its completeness, it frees the soul from its fetters, and once freed, it soars above the daily morass to a state of clarity and bliss. Thomas's love, dedication, and understanding enabled me to endure the tempest of my life, and to reap benefits rather than plunge into despair. Together, I knew we could stand even the thought of death that every ache brought into focus. Thomas's love had made it possible for me to "listen to the hymn of the brook while the tempest roared."

I began slowly to feel intoxicated with life—its daily

routines, its blessed rituals. I felt its pulsating rhythm within me, and I knew my spirit was healed. I knew then that my dormancy would soon be over, but I had to be patient. Time is the greatest healer, so I raised my shoulders high and embarked on the voyage of the life.

3

The Second Fall

Before you are told by a doctor that you might have just a short span left to live, you imagine that you will lead a tremendously exciting life and do everything you ever dreamed of doing. But once the doctor's judgment is decreed, you do not indulge in any extravaganza. All you crave is that simple rhythm of life: to get up, to see your child, to have a cup of coffee, to breathe in the fresh air. You yearn for the ordinary rituals of life.

I found during the four years following my surgery that I yearned most of all for the blessed daily routines. They became most precious to me. I remember one wintery evening when I decided to prepare a fireplace supper. The fire gave me a sense of the essential in life. I was excited, as if it were the first time I had touched a pan. I was intoxicated with joy. "Thomas, Licia, the fire, and Neapolitan songs by Mario Lanza. What else could I want?" I exclaimed.

"You forgot *you*, Mommy," Licia answered. That touched me. My Licia, too, saw beyond the actual supper. She felt the joy of having her mother back. I was grateful for such an evening. Cancer was far away. I glowed in body and spirit.

Such an intensity of feeling, I found, was quite common for me after cancer. Yet, I had to avoid burdening the people around me with my perpetual fervor. I felt I could not impose a steady diet on my family, even though every breath for me became a celebration of life.

The joy of everyday living was heightened. I looked upward more often; I perceived sounds that I had never heard before. One hour of sunshine—what bliss it became. Through my road of doubts, hopes, defeats, agony, and ecstasy, I had acquired that wisdom of the ages to which so many poets aspire—to live day by day, and I remembered Thoreau's words:

> ...I wished to live deliberately, to front only the essential facts of life, and see if I could not learn what it had to teach, and not, when I came to die, discover that I had not lived. I did not wish to live what was not life, living is so dear; nor did I wish to practice resignation, unless it was quite necessary. I wanted to live deep and suck out all the marrow of life, to live so sturdily and Spartan-like as to put to rout all that was not life, to cut a broad swath and shave close, to drive life into a corner, and reduce it to its lowest terms, and, if it proved to be mean, why then to get the whole and genuine meanness of it, and publish its meanness to the world; or if it were sublime, to know it by experience, and be able to give a true account of it in my next excursion. (Henry David Thoreau, *Walden*)

When everything goes well in our lives, we tend to be embedded or suspended somewhere between the past and the future. The nostalgia for the past, the yearning for the future, render us oblivious to the passing day; to the little child who tugs, ignored, on Mommy's skirt while she busily prepares a feast for tomorrow; to the sick we do not visit today, and who are gone tomorrow. We withhold today's love until tomorrow, when we might feel more like giving it.

If we could only listen to children and watch them, we would become so much wiser. A little girl asks, "Mommy, when is tomorrow?"

"Tomorrow is when you wake up."

The child eagerly wakes up in the morning and asks, "Is now tomorrow?"

We are like Camus's Sisyphus whenever we think of tomorrow: there is an endless yearning for it, but never an achievement.

Licia's second birthday was, for me, a victory. Four months earlier, I thought I would never make it. It was such a joy to see her blow out the candles. *How happy to be older*, said her smile, her gleaming eyes. *How happy to be alive*, said her mother's tears.

The celebration threw me into deep thoughts. I contemplated that when we leave the world of beauty and merriness, and enter the world of reality and sadness, we become afraid to blow out the candles. We see ourselves growing older. Our body weakens and our spirit ages. We perceive ourselves as worthless. Instead of becoming wiser with age, we become decadent. The numerous candles on our cake should be a proud sign that life has been good to us.

Those who struggle for survival know how truly great it is to have many candles to blow out.

Every little incident stimulated meditation. In a way, I envied the young mothers who expressed relief in having lunch away from the children; the mothers who couldn't wait for schools to reopen so children would go back. I did not have the luxury to say, "Today, I am busy; I shall spend tomorrow with my child." I could not postpone my living for tomorrow; I had to love today.

Still, I found myself often yearning for the future, even though I tried to live fully in the present. I recall one Sunday after church when we went out for lunch. My heart sank watching the young women—shy, timorous, sitting with their parents. Ours was a college town and they were obviously embarking on a new college experience. How lucky those parents were to see their young ones off to college; yet, they did not know their luck, for time was theirs and life was a matter of fact. I wished and prayed that I, too, would see Licia off to college, but then I thought, "First I have to see her off to kindergarten." I smiled at how easy it is to live for the future even for me, who was constantly bathing in the waters of the present.

My consciousness of time passing expanded to include all aspects of life. Wasting it was, to me, one of the greatest sins. I developed a strong reverence for any form of life, which transcended my own. As a part of the human race, I felt ever embedded in its struggles and its victories. Thus, every life sustained me as every death diminished me. Every cancer death, in a way, became my death; for I was also a new member of this group of sufferers. John Donne eloquently expressed this sentiment in "Meditation 17." I had read this poem many times in my youth, but it had never touched me as it did now that I had tasted the salty waters of life.

> No man is an Island, entire of itself;
> every man is a piece of the continent,
> a part of the main; if a clod be washed
> away by the sea, Europe is the less, as
> well as if a promontory were, as well as
> if a manor of thy friend's or of thine
> own were; any man's death diminishes me,
> because I am involved in mankind, and
> therefore never send to know for whom
> the bell tolls; it tolls for thee.

I also became aware of how much we suffer through misplaced intensity. What seemed of paramount importance to others—a loss of property or the acquisition of material possessions—was for me a triviality. Talk of destroying life, on the other hand, whether through abortion or suicide, saddened me. An empty house burning down was only a property loss—a human life was spiritual loss. Sometimes, what begins as a personal struggle becomes greater than the person, greater than one's own suffering.

Even though I was living at such a high pitch, life had returned to normalcy. The days were filled with a variety of activities. I regularly attended board meetings of the opera guild, where I argued ardently about keeping opera in the original. Once a week, I volunteered at the Beekman Center special needs school, helping the disabled in the Living Center area. I sang in a chorus, and taught Italian in the Evening College at Michigan State University. Most of all, I enjoyed visiting Licia's classroom and teaching the children Italian.

The wound faded, and the rhythm of life resumed. Time is the best cure. It was 1976. Four years had nearly passed, and except for special reminders, such as a cancer death, or a wandering pain, cancer took a back seat. I increasingly immersed myself in projects. I had found a beautiful balance of home life and outside involvement. But suddenly, without warning, the horror of four years ago started again.

It was like a bolt of lightning. I went to see Dr. Leo Mahoney at a cancer clinic in Toronto for a yearly checkup— mammography, thermography, and xerography. The doctor analyzed the test results immediately. I wasn't sent home and told I'd be given the results in a week, as often happens. Appallingly, all the sophisticated tests failed to show the lump. I was fortunate that my doctor insisted on examining the breast anyway; otherwise, I would have gone home happy, but with the enemy lurking inside, once again undetected. Despite modern technology, most lumps are first found by fingertip.

He performed an aspiration, the withdrawal of fluid by suction on the lump, determined that it did not seem malignant, and advised me to check back in with him in a couple months. This was the beginning of July 1976. I returned home to the United States, with that same pessimistic feeling of four years ago. I intuited, again, that the lump was cancerous.

My husband and I decided to see Dr. Schmidt, the surgeon who had treated me before. Again, there were no cancerous signs, but he thought it best to do a biopsy because of my history. Dr. Schmidt suggested a frozen section, followed by the same procedure as before if the lump proved to be malignant. This time I sought a second opinion; I wanted to consult with doctors who believed in other methods of surgery.

I was concerned about undergoing another radical. Other surgeons gave me the pros and cons of each type of surgery, but Dr. Schmidt strongly opposed the method of having a biopsy and then waiting to decide on the kind of surgery. He believed that I should have a frozen section, which would allow him to send several tissue samples to the pathologist for examination, and he would not remove my breast unless there was a malignancy. Again, the procedure he opted for involved aggressive surgery.

I had a long talk with my dearest friend and brain surgeon, Dr. Louis Posada, about the frozen section method, and he confirmed that this is the surest way to detect microscopic cancerous cells in adjacent areas. He used the same method in brain surgery. He assured me that he frequently found the first sample benign, whereas other unsuspected samples taken from adjacent areas proved to be cancerous.

So, I went back to Dr. Schmidt, who ultimately convinced me that his was the safest and most effective way. As it turned out, he was right.

Once again, the week before surgery was hell. This time, I was more fortunate, because my husband's 94-year-old grandmother was with me. We lived this tragic week together. We were the antithesis of each other. She implored for death in exchange for life; I for life only. We prayed that the lump would disappear, and followed a daily routine of checking and rechecking. My mother and my sisters called every day to ask whether the lump had shrunk. I deeply regretted subjecting Grandmother to my suffering, watching her pray continuously, perhaps asking the Lord that she should die rather than I; hoping her death would give me life.

My apprehension about the surgery was different this time. I did not mourn the loss of a breast; I mourned the laborious road I was to travel. Before the first surgery, I feared the unknown; this time, I feared the known. I was no longer an infant in the world of pain, but a mature adult, who doubts her strength to travel the heavy road.

My task now was not to do research at the library, but to prepare my five-year-old, who could not be left asleep this time. She had to witness my departure. I tried to involve her in my suffering; yet, I had to take care again not to overwhelm her. She was so happy about life, and enjoyed her summer days. I saw through her that life flows forward and not backward; one stops to cry, but then moves on. I found myself again suspended between life and death. As I reached out for the ecstasy of life, I saw the cavern of death—I hung suspended between joy and sorrow, swinging from one to the other with great force.

This suspension was especially palpable the day before I went into the hospital. It was my birthday, and we celebrated. Everyone was wonderfully generous with gifts— each one symbolic of our happy life. My family was enormously supportive and tactful. They were worried about my future, but no one wanted to betray their secret fear. The Carlsons too were great. Their presence reassured me that everything would be all right. Licia, cheerful and unaware of my turmoil, played "Happy Birthday" on the violin, and helped me cut the cake.

I could not help but think that this might be my last birthday. I fell back into a now-familiar pattern of thought. I asked myself, "What will the future bring: lots of living, or struggles to survive?" How I longed to grow old beside my husband and to see Licia through the many glorious stages of life. It seemed normal to wish these things. But only God knows the future. Many swimmers never reach the shores of life. They drown as they long for the warm, soft sand of the beach.

The night before surgery, I found myself alone in the same hospital room and same hospital bed, number 2. I insisted that Thomas remain home with Licia. I was not afraid of the surgery. This time, I was involved in writing a fairy tale for Licia about my life—how I met my husband and how she came to us. I wrote it in a childlike fashion and sent it to her so she could read it on the day of my surgery.

In the story, I described our dreamlike existence; our enchanted life together. Thomas was my prince who introduced me to a marvelous kingdom. I was a foreign princess eager to learn everything about my new country, whose humanitarian activities had reached my family and me way back in Italy in 1945. (I still recall the pretty clothes, the medical supplies, and most of all, the delicious chocolates we received through the Marshall Plan.) Ours was a real-world fairy tale, a case of "life imitating art." To complete our dream, we were blessed with a child, a true wonder of nature.

I felt good after I wrote my fairy tale. Whether I lived or

died, I had completed my mission, and were I to die, I would be at peace.

I decided to approach this round without pre-op drugs. I was curious about the operating room, how it looked. I wanted to be fully conscious and alert as I was wheeled down holding my Thomas's hand. That ride on the elevator, how ominous. Why waste that precious time? Most of all, I wanted to say goodbye to Thomas in a clear voice, and with a real smile, so that if I did not come back alive, he would remember me conscious and coherent. I wanted Thomas to see me off au naturel, rather than dulled by sedatives. Wanting to preserve this image for Thomas also helped me not to cave in.

I thought, too, that it would be nice to shake Dr. Schmidt's skillful hand before submitting myself to it, and to thank him for all he had done for me. Whatever happened, I felt he should know that he was the most sensitive, considerate, and concerned doctor I had met in a long time. How could I, then, abandon myself to sedatives, when there was so much to see and feel?

In any case, I did not need the sedatives. I do not profess to be heroic, but having undergone the same surgery before had the perverse effect of reducing the fear and apprehension for which these drugs are designed. It is the déjà vu effect.

As I entered the operating room area, I saw other women parked in the corridor. I, too, was parked there briefly, conscious of us all as fellow members of the suffering human race. I was wheeled into the operating room, where the anesthesiologist was waiting. We spoke about opera, and I began to sing an aria from La Traviata, in which the heroine dies of consumption. The surgeon arrived, wished me luck, and I fell into a deep sleep.

When I woke, the familiar bandages told me that tragedy had struck again. I have a hazy recollection of a nurse with the chubbiest hands. Her voice was gentle and soothing as she repeatedly whispered, "You'll be all right." The soft plumpness of her hands was especially comforting.

I moaned and moaned until I regained full consciousness back in my hospital room. There, I found my husband, our friends, and the surgeon, telling me how very fortunate I was. The lump was not malignant. What *was* malignant was the third sample of microscopic adjacent cells sent down to the pathologist. Had I just had a lumpectomy, I would have been sent home relieved, but with the killer onboard.

I was somewhat comforted that the cancer was detected; yet, I was now stripped totally. I felt tilled, completely, like a field ready to be planted. I had a sweet-sour taste in my mouth—I was thankful that the cancer had been caught in time, but devastated that it had to happen again. I felt an intense sense of loss, the bareness, the desolation of a wasteland. But with the loss came a sense of peace, free for the first time in four years from the anxiety over whether the cancer would spread to the other side. The horror of mutilation was no longer there. In fact, physically, I was more balanced. Now, with both breasts removed, I felt "equaled out." As Thomas said, "Now you can be a flat-chested woman like the flappers back in the twenties."

I did nothing but lie there in my desolation, ready for the seed of life to penetrate my being. There was nothing I could do but wait for life to fill me.

PART II: INTERMEZZO

Life is not a problem to be solved,
but a mystery to be lived.

Søren Kierkegaard

Cancer is for many a way of life—an unsolvable problem, a mystery for both the patient and the scientist. Victory in cancer does not come easily; yet, legions of courageous people fight mightily against the odds. Perhaps what counts in life is not the victory but the struggle. Victory is elusive, ethereal; it can come uninvited, and often, undeservedly. It seems to disappear as fast as it comes. And it can leave us untouched, cold. The struggle, on the other hand, is like the night: heavy, ominous, dark, but it discloses the day if you survive it. This chapter is a glance at how to attack a problem like cancer—everyone's nightmare.

Our strategies for dealing with problems stem from attitudes formed early in life. The method I learned in midcentury southern Italy is simple, perhaps old-fashioned, but it has proven highly effective for me.

I do not have any new formulas on how to live with pain or loss; rather, I revive some old ones from my childhood in my beloved country, where suffering was a daily occurrence and everyone's preoccupation, and consequently, everyone's resurrection. One did not have to suffer a personal loss to be affected. It was enough to partake of the common sorrow.

The funeral processions with the ladies carrying a *braziere*[1] on their heads, the scent of incense wafting into the air, the oratory, the marching band; all these things combined to bring about an emotional release, a catharsis. As a child, I witnessed many of these processions to the cemetery. The music was usually very somber, and brought tears to my eyes, whether I knew the deceased or not. There was a lot of wisdom in those rituals.

I recall a particular episode, which, perhaps more than anything else, taught me how to face the loss of a breast without being destroyed. The home I grew up in was the gathering place for all kinds of family events. So it was natural for my aunt and her family, who lived five kilometers outside our town, to move in with us when their infant child, Lina, fell mortally ill. For four heartsick days, we all stayed by Lina's side and waited, and watched, and prayed in front of the little altar we children had built in a cozy corner of the living room. When Lina's condition did not improve, we began to pray harder and louder for a miracle. Our parents tried to explain to us that Lina's life was in God's hands, and that no one, not even the Pope, could change that. A few hours later, Lina died in her mother's arms, surrounded by her brothers, sisters, and cousins.

---

[1] An elaborate copper pan used for burning coals and incense.

We all felt the cruelty of death. As tangible proof that she was dead, we children touched her cold little hands and stared at the pale, delicate face. Everyone was silent. It seemed we needed a few minutes to acknowledge death, which slipped through ever so quietly.

Lina's body remained in our house for two days, amid flowers, children dressed as little angels, and love. Those two days were entirely organized. There were designated times during the day when we would all gather around Lina and mourn deeply. Usually one person would begin by saying something touching like, "She will not be a comfort to her parents." Then we would all abandon ourselves to tears. Some cried louder, to help those few relatives who stood immobile and dry-eyed. When everyone seemed to have reached a catharsis, Grandmother's soft but energetic voice would lead us into prayer. Coffee and warm milk for the children were then served in the dining room, where we sat in reverent silence. The silence was always broken by the recollection of some funny episode that happened to one of us. We would all laugh with tears until my aunt would announce solemnly: "There is a time to laugh and a time to cry; let us then go and cry, for our Lina is no longer with us."

Since we are all suspended between life and death, we should learn to face suffering openly and honestly. Once we fully acknowledge a tragedy, we must then mourn it thoroughly and systematically, for, to the extent that we live it, we can find consolation and peace. Freud was a genius in this respect: he observed that we have to live our sorrow through. Only then can we begin to thrive.

Coping with loss is essential to our happy survival. Let

us then stop praising people who freeze in the face of sorrow and appear to have everything under control, only to end up in the therapist's office, undergoing their catharsis by reliving the experience. That is going backward. Life, however, flows forward. We must do today's chores, for tomorrow will bring its own. It is important to be timely with grief, as with everything else.

A mastectomy must be mourned, like any other loss, and not shrouded as a mysterious event. I invoked three great principles to help me cope with the loss of my breasts and lead a meaningful life. I knew I had to avoid the temptation to reconstruct things as they had been. Surviving a tragic loss successfully depends not on the expectation that everything will be the same, but the recognition that what has changed ultimately makes no difference in one's outlook and appreciation of life. Values do not change; only their priority and intensity change.

The first principle I found most helpful was the universalization of my problem. What happened to me did not happen to me alone. I am not being chastised by nature or God; I am not being put in a corner like a misbehaving child. If we step back and view our problem from a wider perspective, we will see that it is part of the human condition. To universalize a problem is to do away with the torturous complications that plague us today—guilt, punishment, and a sense of isolation. The "Why me? What did I do to deserve this?" attitude is rendered meaningless.

The mass media spend billions to perpetuate the false image that life is a long summer vacation by the sea. But the reality is, it is our lot to struggle. As Ecclesiastes teaches,

"The rain falls on the good and on the bad." Instead of preaching a life of happiness, we should present life as a succession of storms, whether physical, economical, or emotional, and understand that happiness is not a sustained state, but a glimpse here and there. Like crickets, we must develop feelers to sense the coming of happy moments and enjoy their duration thoroughly. We are so busy building a "future" happiness that we miss those precious moments in the present.

When we universalize a problem, we escape our small milieu and join a greater truth: nature. In nature, we find the rhythm of life, of sorrow, of joy. As part of nature, and like nature, we are perpetually changing. The cold winds of March herald the gentle zephyr of spring. Malaise heralds strength and growth if one accepts the struggle. We are not above nature, but one with nature, and as such, in a constant state of flux.

The wisdom of the trees must be ours. They bow their branches to the strong winds and snow, lest they break. The Inuit, like the trees, obey the law of nature. When they see the storm coming, they do not confront it stubbornly and blindly; rather, they seek shelter in an igloo, and outlive the storm. How wise they are. We, too, must stop and ride out our storms by bending with the wind and by drawing on the reservoir of strength and wisdom in our spiritual igloo. Like a bottomless well, we find that the more we draw from it, the more there is to draw.

Another important principle of great help in dealing with a problem is the law of relativity. It is not enough to understand it in its scientific context; we should know how to apply it to our personal circumstances. For the person whose alternative is to drown, the idea of clinging to a raft for a few days in frigid waters is not unbearable, as it might seem to someone comfortably lodged in bed.

Problems do seem less monumental when viewed in relation to worse situations. What is the loss of a breast in comparison to the loss of a life? I do not underestimate the cruel process of mutilation that, considered in its unrelated state, can be truly devastating. Mastectomy sounds horrible to those who fear being struck by breast cancer—yet, to those of us already in the battlefield, there lurk worse enemies and greater losses. We cannot afford to live in absolutes; they are as damaging as they are specious. Our problem, however dreadful it may seem, has many companions in this world.

Now, it is not enough to universalize and relativize a problem. To stop here is to reach the peak of a mountain and forget to look up. The sense of being close to the unreachable, the exhilaration of having climbed so far, would be lost. The third principle, then, is the spiritualization of a problem. Suffering without meaning is like a dish without salt: insipid and tasteless. It leaves a sense of emptiness and sterility. How do we endow a loss with meaning? We must look at it, and face it with patience, positivism, and good sense.

Since everything is inhabited by positive and negative forces, we are wise to identify the positive aspect of our misfortune, regardless of how minute it may seem. Dwelling on the loss is of no use, for the loss is obvious; we must, instead, focus all our energies on how to benefit from it. My mother would always recite a beautiful proverb when things

seemed hopelessly bleak: *"Non tutti i mali vengono per nuocere."*
Not all misfortunes come to harm us. How true!

Pain is a necessary evil. If handled properly, it can be a source of growth. Pain is, in a way, like winter; it either kills us or fortifies our infant spirit. (I love winters; they make me feel strong. Every ounce of courage and fortitude is called forth on a wintery day. All my inner strength pours out to warm my chilled hands.)

If a meaning can be attached to suffering, then we have won the battle. There lies the real victory. No one likes to suffer for nothing. My war against breast cancer followed shortly after our country's war in Vietnam. The brave American boys who came home were not embraced with the fanfare of the First and Second World War soldiers. Theirs was a return to a bitter country where their efforts were resented. Their courage in battle did not inspire ballads, but evoked disdain from throngs of Americans who saw it as a senseless war.

We need an ideal, a meaning to make our suffering valiant, to uplift it from the daily morass. "It is human to fall, but it is divine to rise," my father used to say when my torment over a scraped knee seemed unbearable. We do have an alternative. We can turn hell into heaven if we have a purpose and meaning. We must develop our inner strength, as a good skier develops muscles and good judgment. A mastectomy patient, too, develops new muscles and strengths, if she chooses to.

These strengths, however, are not easily cultivated in our modern society. Many are the diversions to dull the pain of ordinary living. We are like the child who is given a new toy to make him forget his pain. But as the novelty of the toy wears off, he begins to cry, for the pain is still there. We use myriads of new toys to distract ourselves from our suffering. We grasp for whatever comes to us, hoping that the busier we get, the less we have to face our struggle.

We also live in a fast-paced world, in which problems are far more inconvenient than they were for our mothers and grandmothers. So we tend to ignore problems, and worse still, we don't make time to act upon the signs that herald them. How often do we hear people say, "I have a little growth, but have no time to go to the doctor and have it checked. If it doesn't go away, I'll go next month." Next month comes and the growth is still there and the person is just as busy, if not busier. I wonder whether the modern philosophy of "everything is replaceable" does not give us the illusion that we, too, are replaceable.

We live in an age of instant solutions to newly created needs. Like the rice we buy, we expect everything to be instant. Our motto seems to be: Instant happiness—why not instant suffering?

Unfortunately, suffering cannot be relieved as fast as happiness can be grasped. Sufferings that are shelved leave us unfulfilled, like a brief shower on a hot, humid day. The air feels no more cool and clean. No cosmic catharsis has been reached. Like nature, we need to reach a catharsis in order to clear the air and find new awareness and growth.

Because modern culture does not equip people to successfully deal with adversity, it is imperative that we learn how to cope with the storms of life at a very early age. We must expose our children to struggles in the sanctity and security of the home, and teach them how to find their own balance so that the struggle will not destroy them. Children must develop the wisdom of knowing how far to go. The best way to foster this inner equilibrium is to let them witness adults confronting suffering at home, for the home remains the best-equipped environment for learning.

I still recall vividly the sadness on my mother's face; her anxiety as she clasped me to her breast to comfort me from the pangs of hunger in 1944, when a single loaf of bread had to feed seven people for a whole day. She did not try to distract me from the pain, or pretend that everything was all right. She let us children share her feelings of helplessness, and amid her tears she brought forth a soothing smile. She always ended our little sessions of pathos with a positive remark like: "Thank God we have each other; how could we survive the war without you beautiful girls." How wise my mother was. Even after hours of my crying for a piece of bread, she could still utter such supportive words.

The long evenings reciting the rosary on our knees at home when I was a child were not just prayer, but a valuable learning experience. I recall one particular event when we all prayed, even the feeble old ladies down the street. My father had experienced financial difficulties and my mother and we children were fearful of losing all that my parents had worked for. I am sure God would have answered our prayers even without the children, whose voices faded as the number of Our Fathers grew. Yet, there was more wisdom in those gatherings than I realized then. They taught me that we do not have to be alone in our suffering. Alone we cannot carry the burden of living. Where a person's ability reaches its apex, God's begins. How encouraging to know that there is a greater force than us, a force that will help us cope with adversity.

I also learned that the coming together of family was a remarkable buffer for us children. We had glimpses of the agony even though we did not fully understand it. Like little trees, notwithstanding the protection of the oak trees, we got wet. What a marvelous experience as I recall it now: to feel pain, yet not to have to cope with it alone. I came to know very early in life that while you cannot appreciate the view from the mountaintop until you have been in the valley, the valley is only tolerable when you share it with others.

It is not easy to spiritualize cancer, to give it a higher meaning than its physical torments. It is, indeed, an awesome task, but I know it can be done. Those who hear the hymn of the brook while the tempest roars recognize that not all is lost; that even in the midst of a storm, one has choices. Losing a limb is tragic enough to make one abandon the ship of life, yet there resides in us a strong impetus for survival upon which the mind will naturally concentrate. How comforting to know that we have innate resources to sustain us in the darkest of times.

A mastectomy patient must struggle with dignity, for her story may have as powerful an influence on others as a Shakespearean hero, a Verdi aria, or a Beethoven symphony. We are all actors upon a stage, and many are our spectators. But we do not have to write great books or symphonies to leave our mark.

The way we handle our ship in a storm is our legacy. We can live our last days miserably, or we can choose to spiritually strengthen those around us. We do not have control over how we enter this world, but we do, to some extent, control how we leave it. Like good tourists on a tight schedule, who try to expeditiously absorb all the sublime art of Renaissance Florence, we, too, can do more living in a short time than those who ignore the glory that surrounds them, like the native Florentines who say, "Florence will always be here, and so will we." We are tourists on this planet, not residents of it. Let us do our daily sightseeing.

Immersed though we may be in our struggle, we must maintain our panoramic vision. We cannot change the course of our battle entirely, just as we cannot change the course of a river, but we must find a balance between suffering and daily living. To shelve our sorrow and pretend it is not there is chaotic; to live it to its extremes will kill us. Perhaps we should immerse ourselves in this Life Force and float in it— not try to swim and fight the ocean, but exert ourselves simply to "make the deep, deep sea keep you up."

Nature enfolds us in its rhythm of life and death and resurrection. Living in communion with nature, we can restore that delicate balance within, that safety valve that shuts out stimuli whenever survival is threatened. Being one with nature means respecting its ebb and flow.

Like the Inuit, we must be attuned to nature, to its clues of sanity and wonder, and to its ability to renew itself. Such power of renewal is in every living thing. We, too, have it locked in the sacred chambers of our spirit. We must find a way of unleashing it. Let it pour forth when the tempest roars!

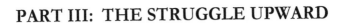

PART III: THE STRUGGLE UPWARD

4

On Visitation

Visiting a sick person is often a trial, for we become preoccupied with our behavior and the effect it may have on the patient. We deprive people of our visits for we do not know what to say, or how to act: shall I be cheerful, pretend nothing happened, cry with the patient, or simply be silent?

Visiting a cancer patient can be especially difficult, for cancer, more than any other illness, tends to illuminate our own finiteness. Thus, a visit with a cancer patient may entail some introspection and contemplation of the human condition. Such reflections can be for some an awakening, for others an unbearable chore better forgotten, or postponed as long as possible.

Those, however, brave enough to step into a hospital room or into the house of someone who has known suffering, must remember that perhaps their presence, more than any words they can utter, is the greatest gift. Visiting a cancer patient is not an occasion for great speeches or a display of joviality. It is an occasion to be oneself; to act naturally and normally. The simplest word, the squeezing of a hand, a tear, an embrace—these are all manifestations that we care, that we are there to acknowledge somebody else's suffering.

After my second mastectomy, I experienced something very beautiful. My friend, Lya, would steal into my room every evening before visiting hours and would sit near me, holding my hand and, absorbed in the most reverent silence, she would watch me doze off. I still remember her lovely features when I close my eyes—her posture of peace is indelibly imprinted on my mind. Then I would wake up, she would squeeze my hand, say a few words, and go home to feed her family. Her tranquility, her meditations, her stillness, and her presence were quieting experiences for me, and a source of strength. Her peacefulness soothed my broken spirit.

What I found most pleasing were the brief encounters. They were as refreshing as the morning dew's beautiful pearly drops. But as the day went on, those pearly drops dissolved, and so did my strength if people lingered. The long visits can be too heavy on a sick person. They drag on and on, until the initial joy of seeing the visitor turns into a struggle to keep one's eyes open. Perhaps I am selfish, but I got annoyed whenever two or three people would come together to see me, sit on my bed facing each other, chatting as if they were visiting together at a restaurant. I repeatedly wanted to say, "Leave the room, and go to a coffee shop to carry on your conversations." I could not be part of that.

Men often feel uncomfortable when visiting a mastectomy patient, for the breast is part of a woman's private anatomy. We think we are liberated, but in real-life contact we can be very Victorian, embarrassed, and shy. We live in a media myth of total sexual freedom and openness, but the truth is that most parents don't parade naked in front of their children, and men don't see topless women every day. In real life, we do preserve a sense of privacy. If one has cancer of the "fingernail," everyone is open and frank; if it is the breast, no one knows what to say. What difference should it make whether it is foot surgery or breast?

I had delightful friends who came to see me. One was priceless as he barged in carrying a freshly baked cookie in his hand, saying: "What is a breast? You look as beautiful as ever. Who cares about a breast?" The nurse standing at the door winked at me and, ready to burst into laughter, left the room. I found Bob's spontaneity very refreshing and even now, whenever I bake cookies, I see him walking into the hospital room with that monstrously big cookie.

Another dear friend came to visit, but he was so nervous about what to say and how to act that he began to ramble on about his life and his retirement. This angered me (though I know his tactlessness was unintentional), for there I was living hour by hour and he had his whole life planned in front of my eyes.

I am not implying that visiting is by any means harmful to a patient. Quite the contrary; it is very beneficial and healthy, for visitors are the only link a patient has with the outside world. It is important to maintain that link, because it speeds up recovery. The patient who lacks this connection may have less desire to join the world outside the hospital, and in turn, her recovery may be seriously hampered. Also, visitors provide a wonderful respite from roommates, nurses, and one's own suffering. Visitors can serve as a vehicle for the patient to voice her frustration, her sense of loss, her trauma. A yoke that is shared is indeed lighter to carry. However, we must keep in mind that a person is in the hospital because he or she is sick and needs rest and gentle stimuli, not exhausting, long conversation.

At home, I found visits much more tiring, for although I felt better, it was strenuous to cope with a busy household. There are more stimuli at home, more sounds to absorb, more joy. Thus, one wears out sooner. Home visits should be shorter than those at the hospital for the first month, because the adjustment back to normal life can seem overwhelming. Young children also resent having to share their mommy with friends now that she is theirs again. And talking at length about your condition with friends is not healthy for the child who, nestled near mommy, absorbs it all. Who can tell what fearful imagining may arise. More time must be spent with little ones to reassure them, and to re-establish the harmony that a hospital stay disrupts. It is a stress to have this delicate mending process interrupted constantly by a ringing doorbell. At home, too, one needs visiting hours, so that uninterrupted rest can take place, and the family nucleus can renew itself.

Do not deprive a patient of the joy of your visit by being worried about what to say. Be yourself; trust your instinct. In this situation, instinct may be our best guide, for we are blessed with timely intuition.

Whatever you do, do not waste time singing the praises of someone after he or she is gone, for that benefits no one. In his delightful book *The Fall*, Albert Camus describes the superintendent of an apartment building. The old man falls sick and is on his deathbed. The tenants hurry in and out of the apartment building, never taking a minute to go see the old man. When he dies, all the tenants pay their respects, each eulogizing the poor old man they had scarcely known or visited in his many years of duty. Let us not be like those tenants—sing the praise and make the visit today, for tomorrow may be too late.

5

On Clothing

What matters in life are the little things; they are the jewels that adorn us with happiness. It isn't the big planning or the grand adventures that fill our hearts with wonderment, but the sweet smile of a child, the passing rays of sun, a kind and loving glance, a dress that makes you feel like a queen.

It is not uncommon for a mastectomy patient, lucky to have survived the storm, to feel this satisfaction and reverence for the small things in life. For her, there are no more ambiguities as to what is important. However, while some of the little things are sources of pleasure, others can destroy that inner equilibrium so earnestly and systematically fought for through her *via dolorosa*. One of these many frustrations can be a new restriction in clothing, especially difficult for a young woman. She is painfully aware that we live in a world in which physical beauty is highly praised and yearned for.

She finds herself surrounded by human beings who strive for physical perfection. But society has defined perfection as that which is not human; that which has no scars, and does not age—that which is coated in plastic, unchanging and forever young—a Barbie.

She is bombarded by mass media that pay millions upon millions of dollars to paint the false picture that she is just a short step from reaching perfect beauty. If you only use this or that cosmetic, you will be transformed from Cinderella into a princess. How can a mastectomy patient compete in this cult of beauty, in this culture of beautiful people?

As a young mastectomy patient, I felt that I could survive almost anything quite well. Yet, there are those pesky things, like little mosquitoes that can so easily disturb the peace. I recall one incident when I found an exquisite dress made of Italian silk. I could not wear it off the rack, for it had to be worn without a bra. Since I was in a designer's shop, the designer agreed to change it to suit my needs. Once altered, the dress lost the sense of freedom it had evoked, but I bought it anyway.

I wore it to a party, and even though I was beautifully dressed, I felt that in comparison to the other guests, my outfit was all too conservative. Many young women there were wearing décolleté necklines that revealed their bosoms. Some of the dresses were not expensive quality, yet were nevertheless sexy and appealing.

I was terribly depressed, and when we got home, I flew into a rage and tore the dress to pieces. My husband stood there, holding my little girl, who, frightened by the outburst, was crying on his shoulder. He comforted her by saying,

"Mommy will be all right; it's just that she is going through a very hard time, and you and I have to help her." I felt my entire philosophy of appreciation for life, my sense of absolute gratitude, going up in smoke. But when the waves of anger subsided, I recognized myself as a very human young woman, who resented the burden of being restricted in what she could wear. I eventually regained my equilibrium and accepted the incident as a normal, common irritation and nothing more.

It is difficult whenever one's freedom is in any way restricted. But as long as you acknowledge it, you can usually bounce back.

The year after my first mastectomy, I became involved with the local opera company. As I resembled the soprano who was singing the title role in *La Traviata* (the opera about a beautiful woman who dies of consumption), the producer asked me to play the soprano's double in the death scene at the beginning of the opera, as the orchestra played the overture. Since I felt qualified in such matters as dying (I had died a thousand deaths the year before), I accepted.

The soprano was staying with us, and on our way home from rehearsal, I inquired about the nightgown I was to wear. Was it décolleté? Was it transparent? You never know how these opera heroines choose to die. After all, they are supposed to be beautiful and sexy. Oh, how I felt the anguish of my body not being perfect that evening. The opera singer described the gown to me. I seemed such a prude. Then I asked about where we would be changing. She indicated that it was in her room, but that others would be present. She was perplexed, and a little annoyed with all these childish questions, and in exasperation, told me she could not understand why a beautiful young woman like me should worry about such things. "Besides," she said, "you act as if you are an invalid!"

An invalid I did feel that evening, and yet, I was proud of myself—that I was facing my problem now in a real arena and not just in my mind. When I finally wore the nightgown, I felt great. It was Victorian and absolutely lovely. The night of the performance, my little Licia, now three, was there. The orchestra began playing the overture; there I was onstage, lying in bed, the doctor coming to tell me that my life is nearly over. I experienced the true drama of death all over again, which in turn infused me with a tremendous sense of rebirth. I also felt very Italian, because in Italy, drama and life are one. And there I was, the embodiment of both. I later learned that my Licia was frightened, and had asked her daddy whether I was really going to die. Perhaps that scene gave her the opportunity to voice her horror from the year before.

Another worry I had to confront was changing in front of other people. Would they be shocked to see part of the scar, or prosthesis, instead of a breast? This fear emerged in another production, the opera *Carmen*. I loved being in it; I am a Gypsy at heart, like Carmen, but I was hesitant about the costume changes. I ended up deciding to go accompanied by a dear friend, who was aware of my fears but insisted I fight them.

The anticipation of the production was very exciting, but I felt a sour note inside. How can I change into Gypsy garb in front of all the female chorus singers? How can I wear those flimsy outfits? Fortunately for me, there were, amid all the décolleté looks, some gorgeous, Renaissance-like costumes. I wore one of those and felt like a true Gypsy in it.

Initially, I was disappointed to be the most covered-up, modest Gypsy. But when the producer instructed the others to look more like me, because of my long hair, my vitality, my flashing eyes, I was more than reassured. It turned out all my other attributes made up for the one thing that was well hidden. In a way, I felt like more of a woman than someone with two breasts, for I had transformed a "deformity" into a victory. I had truly conquered this aspect of the cancer. I felt so proud that I would not have traded my life for anyone's. And on that stage, I felt beautiful. No one could have ever known that I had had a mastectomy by the way I carried myself, brimming with confidence.

The night of the performance, I strutted on that stage, not as someone who has been intimidated by life, but as one who has conquered it. It felt like the renaissance of my life.

It is amazing what a person is capable of in the face of tragedy. You can climb right back on top of the world. This is the beauty and power of us human beings. We have the ability to conquer the unconquerable, to see the invisible, if we only choose to. Let not a disease and all its problems obscure for long this marvelous gift, which is ours alone.

It is normal to demand that we enjoy life. The key is not to cease desiring, but rather not to let the desires destroy us. We are all marionettes at one time or another; the magnificent thing is that we are also the puppeteers. We can take control of those magic little strings, and dance our best dance.

I felt precisely this phenomenon, particularly the first summer after surgery. I wanted so desperately to wear a white bikini. I felt suspended between this desire and the fulfillment of it until one day I pulled the "string" controlling my legs, walked myself to the store, and bought one. Well, my ordeal was not over. How does one hide the prosthesis? I bought a haltered bikini two sizes bigger and sewed a pocket for the prosthesis inside. Then, I made the rest of the bikini smaller, to fit me well. The first day I wore it in public, I made sure my long hair hung on the right side, gently covering it. After a few hours, my "Beatrice" (Licia) pulled me into the water and we both had a wonderful time. A small mark of the surgery was visible, but by that point, I was so deep in seventh heaven, I paid no attention to it.

Take time to take care of yourself. Try to look your best; don't be too introverted or life will pass you by and you will have no one to blame but yourself. Though we strive for perfection, it is healthy to remember that we live in an imperfect world, a world more livable because of its imperfection, a world more human. No one else is perfect, why should you be?

Living is an art. It is not what we have in life that counts, but what we do with it. Like some poor and unknown artist, a mastectomy patient may have to fight harder to survive. Nonetheless, she can still paint beautiful sunrises and sunsets. Look at some renowned artists, how little they had and how much they created. We are all artists in the colony of life. It is up to us to create or destroy. Perhaps after a mastectomy, we transcend the ordinary artist, for we have acquired a new dimension which renders our art more human, more compassionate. Perhaps one has to lose something in order to gain something greater. Nothing comes out of nothing.

6

On Marriage

Let me not to the marriage of true minds
Admit impediments. Love is not love
Which alters when it alteration finds,
Or bends with the remover to remove:
O no! it is an ever-fixed mark
That looks on tempests and is never shaken;
It is the star to every wandering bark,
Whose worth's unknown, although his height be taken.
Love's not Time's fool, though rosy lips and cheeks
Within his bending sickle's compass come:
Love alters not with his brief hours and weeks,
But bears it out even to the edge of doom.
   If this be error and upon me proved,
   I never writ, nor no man ever loved.
(William Shakespeare, Sonnet 116)

The loss of a breast is unique in that it does not prevent a woman from carrying on a normal life, yet it can be so insidious and powerful that it destroys her very being. In this struggle, the woman is dealing not only with herself but with a whole society. For today's woman, losing a breast can be especially traumatic, for she lives in a world that spends millions, if not billions of dollars to perpetuate the cult of the breast. We are caught in a web of sexiness, it seems, where the breast is an overcelebrated erotic part of the woman's body.

I would hope that modern, liberated women have more sense than to believe the myth that sexiness or sex gratification depends on two breasts. As my husband says whenever we discuss breast cancer, a woman who thinks that two large breasts will produce a successful marriage, or the man who thinks his weight lifter's body will make them happy, will soon learn that a particular part or shape of the body really has very little to do with happiness, contentment, or satisfaction in life.

I find it terribly unnerving when a mastectomy patient is asked questions such as, Did you feel you lost your femininity after your surgery? Were you afraid that your husband would not find you appealing? Were you afraid to resume sexual activities? I find the implications of such banal questions insulting to the concept of womanhood. Why should a mastectomy patient feel she is less appealing to her husband? What is she to a man, a mere sexual object to be played with and discarded when she no longer satisfies him, whether it is because of a cancer operation or aging? She is a complex human being who is greater than all her parts. If the breast were such a great attribute to a marriage, why then are there so many divorces, and so much sexual discord among people who have never had mastectomies? If the presence of the celebrated breast does not play a vital part in the welfare of a couple, why should the absence of it create such unnecessary fears?

Whether one is hung up on legs, breasts, or long hair, the truth is, there is no one pleasure that is so satisfying that its repeated experience will continue to excite. As my husband says, physical attraction and physical pleasure are akin to a five-year-old's desire for candy and sweets. It cannot be continually satisfied. One becomes bored with the same thing over and over again. The relationship between two people has to go beyond the physical and emotional attraction, and it matters not whether a man tries to assure his wife of this before the cancer operation or after. If you say it before, she will laugh at you; if you say it after, she will respond, "You are saying that to comfort me." So there is no way we can convince anybody. One has to learn by experience. But, Thomas says, to the extent that you can tell a woman that it makes no difference whether she has lost a breast or not—and he knows—maybe it will do some good. It is not a lesson on how to beat cancer, but on how to live life.

If a man were to leave his wife because she lost a breast, he would not be worth keeping anyway, for such a weak and shallow creature does not deserve her thoughts. If he finds her less attractive than before, he is not worthy of growing old by her side, for he is not attuned to the process of life, with its winters, falls, springs, and summers. He is still a child who has not thrown away childish things.

Most husbands, though, are not senseless children, but loving and wise men, whose fears depend not on whether their wives will still be sexy, but whether their wives will survive the ordeal. The fear of losing a husband actually plagues healthy women who, thank God, have not undergone a mastectomy, more than those who reside in this great vale of tears. It is unfathomable the suffering a man endures in seeing his beloved wheeled into surgery, while he is left outside to the long hours of waiting and guessing: Was it malignant? Did she make it?

I recently heard my husband describe that endless wait in the surgical lounge, and I was moved to tears. So that no woman will ever underestimate the suffering of dear ones in her health crisis, I share with you Thomas's words: "I was confident she was going in for a biopsy, a matter of 20 minutes or so. The 20 minutes passed and nobody called. An hour passed, and then an hour and a half. Still no word from the operating room. It was a sensation, a feeling of walking into the water where gradually it keeps coming up higher and higher to your head. At one point, I began to realize it was a radical. Then it went to two hours, two and a half, three hours. At that point, I wasn't even thinking that we had a radical mastectomy on our hands; I began to worry as to what was happening in the operating room: 'Maybe there are complications. Maybe she is not going to make it at all.' Then I didn't think in terms of cancer, or in terms of losing a breast; I said over and over, 'I hope my wife will come out alive.'"

The battle of cancer is a tough one; it is a struggle that deeply touches every member of the family. When I think of how much my husband suffered, how many hours he spent at my side comforting me and sharing every ache and anxiety, I fail to understand all those silly fabricated fears one hears of. My surgeon, who performed many mastectomies, said that in all his years of practice, he never encountered a man who feared the loss of his wife's breast on sexual grounds.

There are greater concerns for those poor men out there in the waiting room—the fear of a greater loss, the loss of a beloved. For the women undergoing surgery, the fear of dying is too monumental to allow any triviality. The single most important adjustment to be made is not to facing life without one breast or two, but to living with the continuous threat of death.

Thomas and I were so much in love that I never worried about my sexual attractiveness to him. Neither did we worry about our sex life. Of course, one doesn't have a mastectomy and immediately resume a sexual relationship. As Thomas says, there is a period of adjusting to the way the body looks. The two weeks in the hospital are great for this. By the time one comes home to a normal physical type of life, the new body is no longer unnatural, and the sexual relationship picks up from there.

I do not want to negate the presence of sexual fears in women less fortunate than I am. But I resent the implications that such fears are inevitable, and that their absence indicates only that one has not dealt with them. (Perhaps what I resent in America is our constant dwelling on anticipated problems. I recall vividly the POW episode in Vietnam, and how the wives were warned about problems that would occur when their husbands returned. They were so saturated with negative expectations that the poor women were bound to feel concerned if those problems did not materialize; nothing was left to actuality, imagination, and ingenuity.) As a society, we should enlighten people, and not bury them in fears.

The most dangerous aspect of our culture's "breast fixation" is that there may be women who have a lump and try to ignore it because they fear the loss of sex appeal. A woman may naturally fear losing her sexiness before breast surgery, when she is dealing only with the possibility of a loss. But when the actual loss occurs, she has more to struggle with than her appearance. I feel that the fears of not being as sexy as before, or of being rejected by one's own mate, are overplayed and needlessly created by mass media, which constantly bombard us with sex symbols. The woman whose only worth in life is her breast is not real. She's a fabricated image to blind people to the realities of life. Ultimately, the purpose of the sex symbol is to sell things. It catches people's attention, and then they listen to the ads! (This is why advertisers use so many half-dressed models around cars, plumbing supplies, and other very "unsexy" products.)

As Shakespeare said, "Let us not to the marriage of true minds admit impediments." We do control what we let into our life, into our marriage. We must screen our fears; live the real ones and reject the rest. To make a marriage successful is a lifelong task, not an hour's work. We must be the custodians of our relationships and keep everything in perspective. That union which we so celebrated on our wedding day was not only a union of two bodies but also of two minds, two spirits.

Cancer or any other sickness is like a fire. We, crude metals, can become more lustrous and more refined if we can survive the heat. It is through suffering that the greatest insights have been realized, masterpieces created, and loves strengthened. We must remember this in our time of trials and not let the loss of a breast destroy us, for we are far more than a breast. We are that beautiful bow in God's hands from which the arrows of the future are sent forth; we are the inspiration of poets, the Ave and the Eva[1], the Queen of Heaven and the mother of man. We as women are a race: a strong, durable, malleable, and wise race. We must display our strength, our vision—especially in time of loss—not by shelving our feelings, not by being timid, but by being reasonable and wise. As my mother always said to us girls when we inquired about what women are, "You girls give tone, strength, and beauty to a home, to a relationship, and consequently to the world." I truly believe that, and I am firmly convinced that no one will intimidate us unless we let them.

No man will find us less attractive unless we make ourselves less attractive, and that is not a peculiarity to mastectomy patients, but is true for all women. We have control not only over what we eat, or do, but also over what we think. A loss is a loss, whether it is a breast, a beloved one, or the loss of innocence. Those of us who have endured the tragedy of a loss have a responsibility to enlighten others as to its reality.

---

[1] *Ave* (as in Ave Maria), spelled backward, is *Eva* (the Italian name for Eve). In one word, we have the contrast between Mary, the Queen of Heaven, and Eve, the mother of man.

When I was in the hospital for the first mastectomy, my many roommates who passed through for a routine D & C would ask me whether my husband still loved me, whether I was afraid he would leave me. I felt sorry for them, for they did not grasp the meaning of the word love. There are too many young women whose concepts of love and marriage are shallow and distorted. I sincerely hoped the women's liberation movement would fight not only for our economic freedom, but also for spiritual freedom.

We as women are our own worst enemies. We are easily swayed right or left by society's portrayal of what we should think, like reeds in the lightest breeze. To be beautiful, appealing, and tempting is an art that I respect and even practice at times. But it is an art that involves more than physical attributes. They are only the surface of a woman's true being. Beauty is a bonus, but goodness and love are the finer virtues.

Perhaps the real question to grapple with when facing a cancer operation is not, Where do I go from here with my physical loss? but rather, How do I live with the realization that I am not going on forever, that I am suspended now more than ever between life and death? To live with the fear of death is to live a very open and intense life. One no longer plays games with oneself or with others. One meets reality head-on and makes the best of it. All of a sudden, you feel like a tourist in a world of permanent residents. We are *all* tourists, but we live as if we are immortal (it keeps the terror away).

How does this new awareness affect one's life and relationships with others? It can become a real problem to live so intensely day by day; it can place undue stress on a relationship. A woman may begin demanding more of her husband's attention, not because she feels insecure, but because she prizes the moment so dearly that she does not want a day to go by without loving. The fear of dying and of being unable to share her spouse's life can become overwhelming at times. The first Christmas after my second surgery, I was so happy to celebrate being alive that I exhausted everybody with my exuberance. My poor husband, after so many rituals, fell asleep mid-ceremony.

Perhaps it is unrealistic to expect our husbands to have the same survivor's instinct we have, the one which makes every moment count. Although a husband suffers intensely, he lives also with many outside demands that he must answer to. He is involved with two worlds: the world of the home and the outside world. He cannot let one dominate the other; rather, he struggles to keep a balance between the two.

It is exceedingly difficult for a man to go to work straight from his wife's hospital room, to face all the trivia when he has tasted the bitter potion of life. My husband said that after having lived the experience of cancer with me, the problems at work seemed miniscule in comparison. Nonetheless, they were real problems to his clients, and he had to do his best to solve them. I sympathized deeply with President Ford when his wife courageously battled with cancer. He had to bounce from one formidable situation to the other. How hard it must have been to keep a balance, a harmony, between those two very demanding worlds.

It is important for a woman to talk about her suffering, yet it is unreasonable to expect others to respond fully to her plight for very long. Thus, we must not lose heart or become resentful if our family is not there every minute to share each ache and pain. The constant moaning and complaining can be devastating for a relationship. When a man comes home after a long day's work, it is hard to deal with a sick wife!

We need to be wise in our suffering so we do not overburden those around us, for as much as they love us, it isn't their bodies that are sick. Perhaps if one is in horrible pain, it is not a bad idea to take the prescribed painkillers just before the husband comes home, so that some pleasant time may be enjoyed. It is most important during the course of an illness to have flashes of joy and moments of respite. Like a few minutes of deep sleep, such moments can revitalize our tired spirit.

Be vibrant and interested in the world around you, rather than constantly moping and complaining. No one likes to come home to a continually downcast partner. The effort to refrain from complaining is also good for the patient, because it diverts her from her own discomfort and pulls her out of her shell.

I also found that in times of stress, there must be a space between husband and wife, space that allows each to regroup his or her feelings. Men, in crises, tend to act like the Rock of Gibraltar. How courageous my husband was in looking at the wound, in seeing it in its raw state. How brave he was in helping the nurse change my bandages and alleviating my suffering with his wonderful humor. His was a Herculean strength to bathe me, to tend the wound at home without gritting his teeth, to avoid disturbing my peace. Yet, as he said later, rocks do cry; they cry when they are alone. We both cried together many times, but there is a cry, a secret cry, that can only take place in the sacred chambers of one's solitude.

Another realistic fear likely to concern a young mother, more than a woman whose family has flown the nest, is the future of her children were she to die. It is painful but essential to discuss this issue with the husband. A mother may have some special philosophy she wants her children to grow up with. I recall with tears a young friend who was dying of breast cancer, and one of her greatest fears was that her husband would be impatient with their little boy when she was gone. She discussed it with him, and her fears were soon allayed.

The concerns and fears that face a young woman after the loss of a breast are innumerable. The most difficult one for me to deal with and even to voice was whether, if I did not survive, my husband would remarry; and if he did, how he would keep my memory alive in my Licia. The fear of not seeing your children grow up, the fear of not spending old age beside your husband, the fear of not seeing one's life come to a full circle—these are the real fears that we must confront.

Society should help young women who have suffered tragedies to voice these very basic fears and not get lost in the world of trivia, so if life were to end prematurely, they could die in peace and not in despair. All is not lost, for she will dwell in her children's memories. A good husband will not resent honest conversation; instead, he'll love his wife the more for voicing the fears that are also his. We must discuss the future of our children with our spouses, not only for our sake, but also for theirs. If we die, we can still be guiding angels to our young ones.

We must be understanding and patient with the people around us, for they are committed to life and to its many calls. No one can suffer for us, but they can suffer with us. Family and friends can help us deal with our anguish, and even with our fear of death. We must not shelter them from our fears, for they can be a great source of inspiration to us. When one is dealing with life and death, all pretenses cease.

True feelings pour out like a fountain that has been blocked for a long time and suddenly opens to quench the thirst of many. I remember how relieved we were after we discussed death and my fears of not being part of my little Licia's growth or of Thomas's life. We all cried and felt the heaviness of my burden. It did hurt and the temptation would have been to pretend the fear was not there, but by facing it together, we experienced the closeness of our family, the deeply felt sentiments we have for one another.

We experienced our cohesiveness, our fragility, the fusion of three people into one. We saw ourselves as one body with many limbs. When one arm hurts, how can the rest of the body be oblivious to the pain? Physiologically, the body mobilizes all its forces to help the arm heal.

Why shouldn't we mobilize all our family strength to allay fears, to help heal? How natural, if we dispel our inhibitions.

One night, I was so tormented by the thought of death that I could not close my eyes. I finally woke my husband, who gave me a beautiful description of death that calmed me to sleep. He compared death to the host of a party who calls people to join in from the other room. Of course, no one wants to go, for fear of leaving loved ones, and fear of the unknown, of saying goodbye to the only life one knows. Once one enters the other room, however, he or she will discover it is equally enjoyable. It is hard to talk about death, I know; yet, it is inevitable and as such, we must learn to die as we learn to live.

Both my husband and I read an excellent book by Elisabeth Kubler-Ross, *On Death and Dying*, a fine book based on real-life experiences. It bolstered my philosophy of universalization in recognizing that no one who is happy is really ready to die, regardless of age. I was reminded that the fear of death is not only my struggle, but the struggle of all living creatures. If we acknowledge death as an inevitable condition, then we can learn to face it without inducing guilt in those around us.

Children can be very spontaneous about death. One evening as we were driving home, Licia, enchanted by a beautiful sunset, wished that all three of us went to Heaven right then. I felt a chill down my spine over her joy, yet I realized how free children are from life's entanglements. As Christ said, the Kingdom of Heaven is really theirs, and not ours unless we too become like children, free from life's fetters.

After a mastectomy, a woman's greatest desire is to resume life as it was. Yet, can she really recreate the life that she had before surgery? No reconstruction, no cosmetic, can erase the cancer. There is no going back to a "tabula rasa." A host of experiences remain which neither time nor philosophy can negate. The real question is then, Having experienced something that dramatically affects my life, where do I go from here?

We are constantly in a state of flux. Everything changes, including ourselves, whether we have a cancer operation or not. In turn, we must learn to discriminate between those changing things that matter, and those that do not. What an operation like breast cancer can do is expose not only what life's real values are, but what one's values were.

If, for example, wearing a bikini is so important to a woman, and she thinks she can no longer wear it, she will be frustrated. If her frustration continues, she will soon realize that it did not matter whether she would not wear the bikini because of a cancer operation or because she no longer looks as good in it as a 21-year-old. It is, for a young woman, an early lesson in what life is all about. There is a time to laugh and a time to cry, a time to live and a time to die. If it isn't the loss of a breast, it is the loss of a loved one; if it isn't one form of tragedy, it is another.

When one is truly in love, the loss of a breast is inconsequential. A love based on a limb will not survive. Love is an all-encompassing force that will withstand any ordeal. *"Amor vincit omnia"*—a strong relationship becomes stronger after the storm, a weak one will perish. The Biblical comment that he who has will get more, he who has little will lose that which he has, is very appropriate here.

Many marriages are doomed to failure, cancer or no. Perhaps this is wise to keep in mind, so that no one may attribute a marriage failure to the loss of a breast. If suffering cannot keep a couple together, nothing will, for it is in suffering that our togetherness is most felt and needed.

Tragedies instinctively bring us closer to others, for then more than ever do we realize how fragile the human race is.

I have great respect for a man who faces openly and courageously his wife's loss of a breast. He assumes a very difficult task. He wants to be tender, loving, and attentive, but at the same time, he must not make an invalid of her. It is easy for a woman to give up after a cancer operation, and her recovery depends largely on the behavior of the people around her, mainly her husband. His instinct may be to protect his wife from other people's thoughtless remarks, from undue stress and suffering after a cancer operation; yet, he must offer love and not dependency, strength and not weakness, freedom and not bondage. Out of this giving and dedication a greater love is born, a new awareness of each other.

It is a strange, new, and exciting experience to know the power and strength, the tenderness and warmth, the joy and the suffering of loving and being loved. If anything in this world transcends our finiteness and limitations, surely it must be the love between two people. How can we, then, admit any "impediments" to such a union? Whether we love or cease to love is not a reflection on some aspect of the body, but on our inner being. As Leonardo da Vinci said, "The greater the man's soul, the deeper he loves."

7

On Children

The child is father of the man.

William Wordsworth

Children are works of art, and parents are the artists. A child is like a lyre, apparently simple yet complex to the touch. To play it beautifully, one must perfect the art. Parents, likewise, must learn how to handle their human lyres, how to elicit music and not discord. Unfortunately, many children are left to the wind of chance to bring forth fine music. Some are fortunate, despite contrary winds, and make it; others succumb to discord and spend their adult lives seeking the key to harmony by revisiting those childhood years.

Even under the best circumstances, parenting is not simple. It is an awesome task. It calls for ingenuity, stability, love, and above all, good judgment. It is most difficult to love judiciously and to give freely without asking anything in return, to let the children partake of your joys and sorrows without overwhelming them and crushing their gentle spirit. I discovered the true depth of this challenge as my cancer saga unfolded.

I found it very important to involve Licia in my suffering. Yet, I had to be careful not to belabor my suffering. She became a great help to me. It was as if, for a while, our roles were reversed. She informed me. She gave me relief when I was aching with her simple, genuine remarks; she led me to prayer when I was near despair; and above all, she drew me into the simple rhythm of everyday life. Her many demands made me forget my own; her company made painful experiences funny.

The day I bought my first prosthesis, I was elated that I could now wear more fitted clothes; yet, I became morose at the thought of forever having to wear such an appendage. Licia picked up the prosthesis and said, "Mommy, do you want your turtle?" I burst out laughing and hugged her close, turtle and all.

After my first surgery, I tried to maintain some routines. Licia and I continued to bathe together once the wound had healed. I wanted to hide nothing from her. Perhaps I was aiming to instill in her a normal feeling about the loss of a breast. One can lose a breast and still lead a regular life, like the sweet old lady back in Capistrano to whom I used to bring a steaming dish of spaghetti every Sunday. I always volunteered to take the food to her, because I liked her serene countenance, her erect, slim body, and her long wrinkled beautiful hands always gracefully folded. I loved to watch her stretch her hands out for the dish and then lay one on my head and bless me. She always wore black and somewhat blousy dresses. She looked very flat chested to me, almost caved in; but I never inquired about her condition, for she was beautiful nonetheless.

"She lived to be very old, in spite of her two mastectomies," my mother would whisper whenever the fear of death crept into my mind. Then I would see her again in my memories, in her poor, humble setting, and I would be comforted. I can almost still feel those blessed hands on my head.

Poor lady! How much she must have suffered to endure two mastectomies before anesthesia was even discovered. Yet suffering had not marred her face. Her untainted smile was profoundly spiritual. I wanted Licia to grow up with the idea that one can lose a breast without losing oneself. I would often think of her in high school, perhaps studying about mastectomy, and the effect it can have on people; and I would expect her to say, "I don't recall it was so horrible. My mother did not feel that way." I felt very much the teacher, and immense responsibility for my behavior.

Sometimes we forget that we are all teachers. We influence others by what we do and say and how we handle a situation. And handling a situation does not mean repressing the unpleasant, or pretending that everything is laughable. No, we must teach our children how to cry, for only then will they know how to laugh. Kahlil Gibran, a Lebanese-American poet, says that joy is sorrow unmasked. How true! Only after we have tasted the bitterness of life can we really laugh.

Do not fear letting your children see you at your worst. I

never regretted Licia watching me tear up that beautiful silk dress. I felt that she should see me as a normal human being, with all the frailties, sensitivities, and moments of despair that are inseparable from the human condition. Only when she saw me crying could she appreciate my laughter. Yet, it is important that the child observe a conclusion to an outburst like that. She saw me regain my calm, my receptiveness to her love, my appreciation of Thomas remarking how ravishing I looked, and that I was the most beautiful woman at the party. Children must witness not only the tempest, but also the subsequent calm. The strength of the Greek tragedies lies in the fact that at the end, though tragedy has struck, order is restored.

It is critical that we expose children to how we live our sorrow, our frustration, so they will have a frame of reference in knowing how to express their own sadness and anger.

I also consider it essential that children have a sense of spirituality, a belief in God or Supreme Being, in a force greater than themselves or their parents. When a parent is sick, the child's world is threatened. It was most comforting for Licia to pray to God for my recovery. There is so little children deem themselves capable of doing for an ailing parent. To be able to offer their innermost thoughts to God, so their parent may be restored to health, gives them a sense of strength; a sense of control. The child *can* do something.

Also, faith in a benevolent God or spiritual force, an all-loving force, comforts children in their time of stress. I remember Licia's words one day after my first surgery, when she visited me in the hospital: "Mommy, Jesus comes and says, 'Teresa, get up and go to Licia.'" She especially loved the Gospel story of the young boy who was brought back to life.

Spirituality is indeed an insurance investment for our days of need, and we should not deprive our children of such a benefit. I feel disconcerted when parents opt to let their children grow up in a non-religious milieu, so they can later choose whatever religion they like. How can they choose if they have never experienced any type of faith? To live and manage constructively in a world as complex as ours, we must give them more than proteins and vitamins. We would do well to equip them with spiritual awareness so that when the human morass surrounds them, they can soar above it all.

After my second surgery, I noticed that I had acquired the psychology of the survivor. Each day felt like an ode to life, a blessing to be part of Licia and Thomas's world. Each moment was critical for me. Holidays became more charged with traditions, rituals, and exchanges of happiness. The first Christmas after my second surgery affirmed my rebirth. I felt like a child again, strong and reinvigorated. I wanted Licia to taste the joys of my childhood by concentrating on the real Christmas spirit, the nativity scene.

Licia, her little friends and I went into the woods to find moss, driftwood, and branches to reconstruct the village of Bethlehem. On Christmas Eve, the candlelight procession around the house, the lengthy supper with its traditional 13 dishes, the caroling—all manifested my intoxication with life. Cancer was in the past; there was no scar on me—only a zest for living. Like the tourist who, on his last day of travel, wants to snap every picture possible, I was anxious to imprint on my child's mind pictures of what I was made of.

That Christmas Eve, I was certainly intensifying everything. I failed to see life through Licia's eyes—simple but real. It is easy for a parent to unwittingly overwhelm the child by making everything significant. Children most often function on a simple sonata. I, on the other hand, found myself functioning mostly on the Fifth Symphony. After cancer, one is forever suspended between life and death, and the awareness of death tends to reinforce life. It often seemed quite burdensome to feel so much at such an early stage in life.

Children need frank, precise answers, yet not intense ones. Licia once asked me why we couldn't have any more children, and I answered that my life could be endangered. She quickly interjected, "You mean, you die?" I said that could happen, so she gave me a hug, and she ran out to play, happy as ever.

I discovered that at age six, she really did not understand the problem as well as I had thought she did. After my first surgery, Licia was only 17 months old, and I continued taking baths with her, maintaining the same lifestyle we had had before the surgery. As the years went by, she noticed my prosthesis, and often she held it and called it a "turtle." Yet, despite all this relaxed exposure, she came back from kindergarten one day, saying that her teacher had had the surgery I did. The teacher's arm hurt. Licia had not associated my suffering with the loss of a breast.

How wise children are! They seldom overload their circuits. They have a great sense of how much they can absorb. Just as the typical child does not sit at the table and overeat, so she does not burden herself with more details than she can handle. I discovered this one day when I pulled Licia away from the swings quite hurriedly. On the way home, I explained to her how sorry I was to tear her away in the midst of playing with her friends. I went on and on. She turned to me and said, "It wasn't that bad, Mommy." She accepted the interruption more readily than I did.

As Licia got older, I felt she needed to see other women who had not had mastectomies. She needed to realize that Mommy is not the norm, that she did suffer a loss. I had Licia take swimming lessons at the university, where I was pleased to see her change in the same room as her instructor. I wanted her to grow up with the proper attitude and not to be scared when she started to develop breasts.

My family and I participated in a Canadian Broadcasting Company program on breast cancer, and Licia of course watched the program with us. Her reaction to seeing a woman who had reconstruction was that I shouldn't have it done, for she liked me the way I was.

Sometimes, we fear that children will be shocked if they see us after a mastectomy. If handled properly, it should not have any adverse effects on the child. If the mother is insecure, however, and tries to hide herself when she changes, then the child will infer that mother is hiding something terrible.

Young children often ask where the breast went. I found this the toughest question of all. I told Licia that it went to Heaven. I was very careful to avoid saying, "It was removed because it was sick," as I did not want her to think that every time a part of her was sick, it would be cut off.

With very young children, it is wise to take them with

you when you check into the hospital. I really regret leaving my daughter asleep the first time. Poor child! She must have thought I had disappeared. Had she seen me in the hospital room, at least she would have had a mental picture of where I was. Luckily, I had bought a book by P.D. Eastman called *Are You My Mother?* before I went in. I found out later that she wanted my mother-in-law to read her the book continuously. Licia identified with the little bird that came into the world and saw no one in the nest, so he set out to find his mother. Five years later, Licia brought the book to school one day, and told her classmates how she felt about the story, and how she identified with the little bird.

At the time of my second surgery, Licia was already six years old. She was more mature, although the day of my surgery I saw to it that she read the fairy tale I wrote for her. One does not have to write fairy tales for their children, but a little note, a card, or something personal is advisable so the child will not feel abandoned.

This brings me to a point that I really feel strongly about. What does the child do on the day of his or her mother's surgery? I experienced with Licia that children have to be allowed to live their sorrow. They should not be taken to the circus or anywhere else if they do not want to go. They see everyone around them at home feeling tense and apprehensive, and they should not be sent away or shut in a room. Children must be allowed to cry just as they are allowed to eat. It is their right. They are members of the family, and as such, need to partake of the sorrow, or they feel terribly rejected. Also, people around them must be told how to treat the child. Adults should not try to allay the child's fears by stuffing candies into her mouth; they must acknowledge the child's apprehension, and should not try to distract her.

I recall an episode I once witnessed at the barbershop. A little boy was having his hair cut by a barber who used huge electric clippers that made a loud noise. The boy was terrified and began to cry. His mother kept popping candies into his mouth, instead of acknowledging his fear and asking the barber to use smaller scissors.

The need in children to live their sorrow is intrinsic; thus, we cannot divert its course. Perhaps the reason we try to distract them from suffering is that we feel inadequate when they cry. We become insecure and frightened. But children must be allowed to live their tragedies, so they can accept them. They, too, need to universalize their suffering. Children are very good at finding a book or a situation to identify with. They do it naturally, but only if we let them.

On the day of my first surgery, my dear neighbor later told me, Licia sat on the rocker and rocked herself. JoAnn, thinking that Licia needed comforting, picked her up and held her close. Licia took her by the hand and led her to the couch. Licia returned to the rocker and lullabied herself until I came out of surgery. Perhaps even children cannot share their deepest feelings at times.

The second surgery led me to a new awareness of children. I enjoyed my child so much that I became like the grandmother who slows down with children, and consequently, perceives more in their actions than the fast, energetic mother with pressing deadlines to meet. I could distinguish between what mattered and what did not.

Children need the attentive wisdom of grandparents, yet they also need the strong hand of the parent. I found it hard at times to keep a balance between these two roles. I considered myself blessed to witness another day in Licia's life, and I felt a great need to emphasize the beautiful. Yet, life has many aspects, and children need to learn how to manage a normal day.

The metaphor of the river helped me immensely. I thought of Licia's life as a river that flows forward and not backward. As such, I could not keep her from continuing her course. She could partake of my joie de vivre, yet she could not live it as intensely as I did. She was not I, neither was she mine. She was, to me, a myriad of things: a teacher, who taught me how to laugh while exercising; my vision of Heaven when the slopes of Hell became unbearable to climb out of; and my guide in the return to normalcy, for she was my everyday joy.

Kahlil Gibran's *The Prophet* includes a beautiful passage on children that encouraged me often when I was in doubt:

> Your children are not your children.
> They are the sons and daughters of
>   Life's longing for itself.
> They come through you but not from you,
> And though they are with you yet
>   they belong not to you.
> You may give them your love but not
>   your thoughts,
> For they have their own thoughts.
> You may house their bodies but not
>   their souls,
> For their souls dwell in the house of

tomorrow, which you cannot
visit, not even in your dreams.
You may strive to be like them,
but seek not to make them like you.
For life goes not backward nor tarries with
yesterday.
You are the bows from which your children
as living arrows are sent forth.

Let your bending in the archer's hand
be for gladness;
For even as he loves the arrow that
flies, so he loves also the
bow that is stable.

This passage became my gospel in living with Licia.
When I read it, I felt free and ethereal, and consequently,
worried less about the technicalities in my daily relationship
with Licia. The last sentence of Gibran's poem was especially
comforting, for he who loves the arrow also loves the bow. I,
too, was a child in the eyes of God, a child in need.

The beauty of children lies in their ability to make us feel
like children again ourselves. They are, for us, an inspiration.
We strive to be like them, yet we must at times inspire them.
It is an awesome task, but the greatest of all.

8

On Medical and Cosmetic Decisions[1]

Our world today is an exciting one; we are constantly bombarded with knowledge. It is difficult to keep abreast of all that is happening. We in the United States are perhaps the best-informed public in the world, not only because we are a people of "leisure," but also because we have the blessed freedom to read, choose, and hear whatever we want. Yet, an informed public has also a heavier burden to bear, for with knowledge comes responsibility. We are called on every day to make responsible choices; even going to the supermarket can become a battlefield of choices and responsibility. One has to be a chemist to decipher what each can contains, and what might impair health.

---

[1] The cancer landscape has vastly changed since the time of writing. This chapter paints how the landscape appeared to me then, in the 1970s.

The problem of choices becomes more critical when we deal with health issues, since in medicine, "a little learning is a dangerous thing," and ignorance is no bliss but can cost a life. For a woman who has just discovered a lump, being faced with so many philosophies on how to proceed can be very traumatic. It is hard enough to accept the reality of having discovered the lump, much less to discern which school of thought is better than the other.

This is the time to confer with several surgeons and to discuss frankly how you feel, to voice your confusion, and to ask for statistics on the various methods. Through my consultations with several doctors, I learned that there are two kinds of surgeons: (1) the private practitioner, and (2) the university, academic surgeon. Private practitioners tend to be more conservative; they usually practice the method that has been used for a long time. They are apt to change only when a new method is proven. The academic surgeon, on the other hand, tends to be more experimental, to use newer methods, even though they have not been confirmed by research.

A major breakthrough in cancer has been in the field of pathology. Pathological reports are increasingly more complete, more informative. It can now be accurately ascertained what type of cancer is present, whether it is infiltrative, non-infiltrative, etc. Such information can determine the extensiveness of the surgery.

There was a tremendous controversy among surgeons at the time of my ordeal as to how breast cancer should be treated. Some surgeons had discontinued performing radical mastectomy in favor of partial mastectomy, for they believed there was no acceptable evidence that radical surgery prolonged survival. Even though I was well aware of this controversy, I felt more comfortable with the conservative method.[2]

Many factors enter into the decision regarding what kind of surgery to have if cancer is detected. It is important to be as well-informed as possible, but reading a book or an article on cancer should not lead to overconfidence, stubbornness, or finally, to grave mistakes. We are dealing with a major killer, and not with the common cold. The doctor who says we caught it all by removing the lump or the breast is just as blameworthy as the one who indiscriminately says, "Let us remove it all immediately."

Cancer is too complex an enemy to be treated by one method alone. Surgery may only be the first step: radiation, chemotherapy, and other methods may be needed as a follow-up. One of the advantages of going to a cancer clinic is that doctors there tend to be more adventurous and willing to try the latest discoveries. I learned four years later that perhaps I should have had chemotherapy, as two-thirds of my lymph nodes were found to be cancerous.

It is important to know the most current options in

---

2 In 1979, thanks to many activists and scientists, we saw an end to the Halsted radical mastectomy. My surgeon warned me that if I survived I would see the end of it, but he wanted me to know that he did the best he could with the knowledge he had at the time. I reassured him that I am an existentialist and that if we do things *à la foi* (in good faith), we have no regrets. I have no regrets. I feel blessed to have survived cancer for 40 years. I am thankful that women no longer have to face the mutilation I experienced, and happy that new techniques like lumpectomy exist, followed by more effective radiotherapy and chemotherapy.

treatment, but it is just as important to know oneself. One must be like a captain in battle. The best war strategies are planned in known territory, and with as much knowledge as possible about the enemy. A woman has to examine her territory, her personality, her ability to endure, her strength in living with a decision. She must work out all her fears and doubts before she can agree to a particular type of surgery. After surgery, there is no time for self-pity. A new, long road ensues for those lucky enough to see the rainbow after the tempest. It will be too late to regret past decisions.

I was a young woman, and to me the breast meant much, yet not enough to jeopardize my life. There was so little that could be done with cancer. I did not want to lose the slightest chance of survival, so I opted for the radical mastectomy. As a young mother, I had a responsibility to my family in my choice of surgery. It certainly was my body, my life; yet, I felt deeply the duty to stay alive. My life belonged equally to me, Thomas, and Licia—but not to my physical appearance.

Granted, the cosmetic aspect may be more important for some than for others. I am fully aware that a woman's self-image will play a significant role in her dealings with her family, yet I am confident that anyone who survives cancer will emphasize her sense of rebirth rather than her loss.

Much is available for a mastectomy patient in the way of prosthesis. There is one on the market that feels so real that its weight shifts naturally as you turn. Mine shifted so much one day that, as I was bent down gathering flowers, I found it in a flowerbed. I picked it up, laughed, and proceeded with my flowers. Plastic surgeons can reconstruct a silicone breast to replace the missing one. A luxury type of prosthesis is a molded duplicate of the remaining breast, available thanks to Dr. Dennis Lee of Ann Arbor, Michigan.

I cannot stress enough the importance of preoperative preparation of both oneself and the family. For the woman who firmly feels she must have a reconstruction (and there are some beautiful models whose jobs depend on it), or for any woman to whom the disfigurement would mean unbearable torment, it is advisable to speak with the doctor about it. I learned only later that after a radical mastectomy, reconstruction is impossible. I was upset about that and wished I had been aware of it before. Eventually, of course, I was convinced I would have taken the same route, knowledge or no.

I am thoroughly intoxicated with life and I feel blessed to be here today to share my experiences with you. What I want to tell you is this: be prepared, be knowledgeable, but most of all, be wise. Please do not walk to the doctor, but run. Run to the doctor, and if he says your lump is nothing, run to another who will follow a medical procedure and not send you home to watch it grow. What we have in our favor is early detection. Cancer will rarely, if ever, cure itself. We must not ignore the signs, though the temptation is great. The first reaction is to ignore it, as if we are talking to the child in us: forget about it and it will disappear. Often we find ourselves telling children, "Don't think about it and it will not hurt." Cancer of the breast does not hurt, thus it is doubly easy to forget about it. Unlike the child for whom such oblivion is happiness, for a woman it may be disastrous. If you notice any symptoms during your monthly examination (and don't forget to check your breasts after each period), do run to the doctor.

This is part of our mission, but not the end. Don't make my mistake, and wait for a sunburn or a cold to send you back to the doctor. You may need to insist on further testing. Sometimes it seems the numerous ads directed at patients should be directed at physicians. According to statistics, most lumps are discovered by patients, and some are dangerously neglected by doctors.

In this day of medical-technical advancement, a biopsy is not a complicated procedure. Another quick method available is aspiration, by which a physician can determine whether the lump is cancerous or not. There are many other tests like mammography and xerography, which are excellent means of breast cancer detection using X-ray. Another test available, thermography, detects areas of increased heat emission from the breast tissues. However, thermography is considered only an important aid to diagnosis and not a cancer-detecting procedure. Malignant tumors do emit excessive heat, but so do other non-malignant conditions such as infections and inflammatory reactions.

Another problem I feel is very important to discuss here is one that faces young women. Having cancer at an early age is tragic, because many women may not have a chance to complete their families. The inability to bear children can be excruciating for a young woman. She may be tempted after a mastectomy to find a physician who deems it is safe for her to have children, and it is not hard to find one. But she must be aware of other philosophies on this subject. Some doctors believe that during pregnancy, the hormonal activity tends to reactivate the cancer. Radiation treatments may also adversely affect the fetus, and result in a strong possibility of deformed children.

What does one do? Another horrible dilemma must be faced. I struggled with it for a long time. Although my desire to have children was very intense, my commitment to life was equally strong, and I did not want to jeopardize it. I was sure, however, that if I were to become pregnant, I would not destroy a life to save mine. Thus, more and more complexities arise in a seemingly endless spiral. In spite of them all, there is nothing greater than life, for it is in living that we realize our strength and our weakness, our capacity to struggle and our vision to survive.

Do not let my tale discourage you. Rather, let it show you the depth of living, your ability as a member of the human family to taste both the bitter and the sweet, the finite and the infinite. May you be spared all this suffering, but if this is not to be, let your suffering flow out from the sacred chambers of your heart and encompass us all, for it is in giving that we receive.

PART IV: CODA

9

Incipit Vita Nova[1]

Those of us who believe in God or in a Supreme Being are bound to question God's mercy at times during the struggle with cancer. The question most often asked is "Why me?" The answer perhaps lies in the wisdom of Ecclesiastes. The rain falls on the good and on the bad, the rich and the poor. Sometimes, however, this observation is not enough to calm our anger, and in our helplessness against cancer, we may feel the need to attribute our suffering to something or somebody.

The terror of cancer is that we feel powerless, for we do not know how to control it. Since we are rational beings and like to be dominated by logic, we seek a reason for our suffering. When all our human resources fail, then perhaps

---

[1] A new life begins

we turn to God and ask, "Why are you, oh God, tormenting me with this ailment?" It is hard to believe that a loving Father would afflict us so.

Our bodies are very intricate and as such, they are susceptible to failure or, in the case of cancer, to invasion by uncontrollable organisms. We are part of nature and therefore in a constant state of dying and renewal. As one part of us dies, another comes to life. The cold winds of March herald spring, just as malaise heralds strength and growth.

The Inuit show us the fortitude they derive from nature in their struggle with a force at times far greater than themselves. Their sculptures reveal to the touch the solidity of iron and softness of silk. A weak hand could never have created them. The streamlined form communicates to the viewer a sense of peace and direction, and the subtle vision of their maker. To achieve such tranquility in sculptures, how many blizzards the artist must have endured.

The blizzards of cancer are many and at times unbearable. Yet, if we can accept this as part of the human condition rather than chastisement from God, then we can, through divine providence, ask God to help us find in our suffering a sense of direction, a sense of growth toward a better understanding of ourselves and of the world around us. God can help us to spiritualize our suffering, to rise above the morass of daily living so that we can build on the ruins; so we can gather rather than scatter. He is the creative force in us and He can enlighten and help us turn hell into heaven.

Without divine providence, it is difficult to soar above the murkiness of terrestrial living. But divine providence does not fall upon us unexpectedly and uninvited. We must be open to it and, above all, vigilant to recognize it when it comes. There is a proverb heard regularly in Italy: "*Aiutati che Dio t'aiuta*"—God helps those who help themselves.

A well-known writer and the mother of brilliant children told me that when she had her mastectomy in the 1960s, she felt very alone. She did not believe in God, in a force greater than us, and she envied deeply the other women in the hospital who could spiritualize their suffering. Hers remained at the human level, a mutilation of her body, a destruction of her spirit. How sad she told me it was for her. Religion is, indeed, a foundation for dark days like the ones after a mastectomy.

I feel very strongly that we do an injustice to our children by not preparing them spiritually as well as physically and mentally for life. What will they do when the storm strikes? Will they know how to build their igloo and outlive the storm? As parents, we cannot protect our children from the storms of life. We can only teach them how to cope with the turbulence.

We must be as vigilant of our spiritual welfare as of our physical welfare, so that the blizzard will not catch us unprepared. As my cancer saga unfolded, those same knees that once knelt on the cold tiles of my home in Italy would kneel on the soft bed of the hospital the night before surgery. How frightened I was—I, who used to faint at the sight of a hospital as a child. (Of course, Italian hospitals do stink of antiseptic—a smell that permeates the hospital from its entrance to the surgical lounge—no smell of coffee or freshly baked treats like American hospitals.) After I prayed, I felt as if a heavy burden had been lifted from me, and I began to read a book by Pierre Teilhard de Chardin, *The Phenomenon of Man.*

I was comforted and profoundly moved by Teilhard's optimism. He writes that despite the existence of evil, one can truly see in the universe a sense of direction, a direction toward the "Omega Point" (the supreme level of complexity and consciousness). But in order to experience this direction, we must pause from the march of daily living and let the world around us fill our being with strength and vision.

Today, perhaps more than ever, we are caught in a world in motion. We live at such a fast pace that we are easily swept into a whirlwind of activities. We thirst for experiences to fill our days. To stand still is considered bad—to be in motion, to bounce from one experience to another, becomes a compulsion. We can be so preoccupied with ourselves, our successes or failures, that we almost suffer from a linear vision. We tend to either look forward to success or backward to failure. We do not, generally, look up toward God. That may be simple to imagine, but when one is caught on a treadmill of circular motion, it is very difficult to break the vicious circle. What an illness or any form of serious suffering can do is break this circle, free you from its entanglements, and compel you to take a good look at what life is all about—namely, meaningful relationships with God and with others. When all else fails in life and one is standing on the verge of chaos, it is hard to envision anything more important than a relationship with God.

One does not have to wait for a catastrophe to feel the power and presence of God. It is only necessary to step back from the clamoring world, to stand still, silently, and listen. After my second surgery, I had a beautiful experience. Together with my dear friend Ardis, I went to a retreat in a most inviting place: The Portiuncula in the Pines, a monastery outside of Lansing, Michigan.

As we entered the Portiuncula, I was struck by its heavenly peace. Nature around us appeared in all its glory: tamed, manicured, splendid. Like a bride in her white garments, radiant in countenance, she invited us to enter her kingdom. Everything was fused in a perfect harmony—the inner warmth of the house and the outward serenity of the pines. I was oblivious to everything, yet I felt everything. The apple trees, the birds, the well-rounded hills, all spoke of peace, of God. My cancer seemed to have been wiped away. I saw only the towering pines, their lower branches touching the ground, their lofty bodies outstretched toward the sky. They all spoke of love, of harmony. Under their tutelage, on the soft ground, grew their seedlings, speaking of tomorrow. They too, someday, will be as big and as strong. They, too, will sing with outstretched arms hymns of praise and glory to God. Not far from the seedlings lay the pinecones—brown, withered, yet containing within them the seed of life. There, all in one, under the same tree I experienced in a single breath life and death, one united with the other, to form the whole. I thought of my little seedling at home, and hoped that I, too, like the giant pine would live long enough to give her shelter.

That vision, that supreme moment, will remain with me always. James Joyce called a moment like that an epiphany: an incredible heightening of the senses, and a powerful feeling of oneness between nature, human, and God. (The three so often seem to go their separate ways.) Boris Pasternak, the Russian novelist, called this moment of vision "free time" or "living time… that pure interval in which one glimpses real, brimming life, like the life of trees and animals."

It was euphoric to be there under those majestic pines; I, like the little seedlings, felt sheltered from the tremendous forces of life and death. I felt very much at peace. My worldly cares, my yoke, seemed lighter. The obsession of the world was far away. I could truly understand the Apostles' yearning to pitch a tent on the mountain during Jesus' transfiguration and stay there. The peace, the joy, must have been overwhelming. Like the Apostles, I wanted to stay there, where everything pointed toward the "Omega Point," which seemed to me closer than ever. I felt as if I were climbing the mountain of Paradise, enveloped by a radiant light. This time nature was my guide.

It can be difficult to experience one's spiritual strength and depth in a setting permeated by worldly chores. A few days in ascetic surroundings will nourish our spirits and bring us closer to a vision of God. As Teilhard writes in *The Divine Milieu*, "It is throughout the length and breadth and depth of the world in movement that man can attain the experience and vision of his God." Sometimes we must stand still so that the universe in motion will fill our spirit with the power of God.

"Be still and know that I am God."

Afterword

I met Teresa on the evening of her 44th anniversary with Thomas. The two eternal companions had just set off on a romantic walk when Thomas got involved in a discussion with neighbors, serendipitously freeing Teresa to join me on my mother's porch swing. We immediately connected over my background in philosophy which I shared with her daughter, Licia, our common histories of living in Canada, and our mutual love of writing. She was looking for an editor to revive a manuscript she had written over 30 years ago about her inspirational experience with breast cancer, and I had just finished editing my last project for a dear friend who was coincidentally starting treatment for his own cancer—it seemed like providence.

Teresa was soon engrossing me with her epic tale. After she was featured in a documentary on breast cancer entitled "Four Women" on the CBC series *The Fifth Estate* in 1978, Teresa's manuscript had attracted the attention of a large publisher. She was a few short steps from signing a book deal, but there was one catch. The editor stipulated that a sex scene would need to be added. The heartrending story, the operatic prose, and the wisdom unique to one who has lived the extremes of both beauty and pain, colored vibrantly by the optimism of youth—these, the publisher deemed, were not enough. Here was the very media-perpetuated obsession with sex that Teresa criticized for needlessly compounding the trauma of mastectomy patients, the submission to which was now being demanded of her if she hoped to publish. As important as her message was, and as many as its beneficiaries would have been, the condition was unacceptable. It went against everything she stood for.

So Teresa showed the editor to the door, forwent the book deal, and the manuscript was sadly tucked away. Until, in 2008, Teresa was tragically struck once more by cancer. Diagnosed with a very rapidly progressing non-Hodgkin's lymphoma of the stomach, she began a harsh course of treatment, including chemotherapy for the first time. Turning back to her manuscript for strength, she found it in abundance.

Though she didn't have the energy of the 29-year-old who conquered the first bout, the parallels were unmistakable. Rather than immersing herself in opera and other projects, Teresa turned to nature. Drawing on the healing, restorative power of the monastery pines, Teresa went to work to create her own sanctuary, in the form of a beautiful Japanese garden, reaping the natural bounty just outside her home. The order, the simplicity, and the peace of the garden provided a balance to the utter havoc and ugliness of battling cancer.

As for Teresa's Beatrice—her inspiration on the journey from hell to heaven, which young Licia had once embodied—the role was passed down from mother to child. Licia's son, Julian, would sit with his grandmother in her Japanese garden, lovingly touch her bald head after chemo had deprived her of her beautiful long black hair, and motivate her every day to fight to live. Teresa was reminded once again of the "simple but mighty healing power of a child."

Healing became not only a full-time job, but an art. To the support garnered from her manuscript, Teresa added several new strategies. She discovered that the best approach to confronting such a formidable opponent was to micromanage. Rather than allowing the immensity of chemotherapy to crush her spirit, she held her focus on one day at a time; one task at a time; one treatment at a time. Invoking the power of imaging, she would speak to the cancer cells and inform them that they were not welcome, open the windows, and visualize them with suitcases making their exit. The job of healing involved also reading as many pertinent books as she could get her hands on, close attention to diet, and limiting her visitors to only those with a positive attitude. Aware of the powerful mind-body connection, she would have regular conversations with her body, assuring it she would protect it, fight for it, and do it right by eating well. She took control where control seemed impossible, and refused to allow herself to become a victim.

With nature and child as her guides, a tenacious commitment to mastering the art of healing, and the support system that any major illness requires, Teresa conquered cancer once again. She knew that if her words could encourage one other cancer patient, if her experience could enlighten a single loved one caring for a patient, she had a duty to make every effort to reach them.

We are so fortunate to have arrived at a time in which Teresa can publish her story on her own terms. Like all else in her life, it is with integrity and beauty, with style and nothing but class.

Nivi Nagiel

April 2013

CPSIA information can be obtained
at www.ICGtesting.com
Printed in the USA
FSHW011921220919
62274FS

9 780988 230026